Understanding
TYPE 2
DIABETES

First published 2013
This edition published 2014

Exisle Publishing Pty Ltd
'Moonrising', Narone Creek Road, Wollombi, NSW 2325, Australia
P.O. Box 60–490, Titirangi, Auckland 0642, New Zealand
www.exislepublishing.com

A CiP record for this book is available from the National Library of Australia.

ISBN 978-1-921966-20-0

Designed by Tracey Gibbs
Typeset in ITC Cheltenhem Std
Illustrations by Mark Roman
Printed in Shenzhen, China, by Ink Asia

This book uses paper sourced under ISO 14001 guidelines from well-managed forests
and other controlled sources.

10 9 8 7 6 5 4 3 2

Disclaimer
This book is a general guide only and should never be a substitute for the skill, knowledge
and experience of a qualified medical professional dealing with the facts, circumstances
and symptoms of a particular case. The nutritional, medical and health information
presented in this book is based on the research, training and professional experience of
the author, and is true and complete to the best of their knowledge. However, this book
is intended only as an informative guide; it is not intended to replace or countermand
the advice given by the reader's personal physician. Because each person and situation
is unique, the author and the publisher urge the reader to check with a qualified
healthcare professional before using any procedure where there is a question as to its
appropriateness. A physician should be consulted before beginning any exercise program.
The author, publisher and their distributors are not responsible for any adverse effects or
consequences resulting from the use of the information in this book. It is the responsibility
of the reader to consult a physician or other qualified healthcare professional regarding
their personal care. This book contains references to products that may not be available
everywhere. The intent of the information provided is to be helpful; however, there is no
guarantee of results associated with the information provided. Use of brand names is for
educational purposes only and does not imply endorsement.

Understanding
TYPE 2
DIABETES

→ Fewer highs → Fewer lows → Better health

PROFESSOR MERLIN THOMAS
Baker IDI Heart and Diabetes Institute

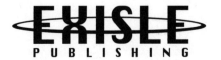

EXISLE
PUBLISHING

Professor Merlin Thomas is a clinician scientist working at the Baker IDI Heart and Diabetes Institute. He works extensively with patients with diabetes and their doctors, as well as performing research in experimental models of diabetic complications. His work aims to identify new targets and advance new treatments to prevent, reverse and retard the development and progression of diabetic complications. He has written over two hundred papers, book chapters and books on diabetes management. His work on diabetic complications has received both local and international recognition including the Victorian Premier's Award for Medical Research.

Baker IDI Heart and Diabetes Institute is an independent, internationally renowned medical research facility. Their work extends from the laboratory to wide-scale community studies with a focus on diagnosis, prevention and treatment of diabetes and cardiovascular disease. The Institute's mission is to reduce death and disability from cardiovascular disease and diabetes; two highly prevalent and complex diseases that together are responsible for the most deaths and the highest health costs in the world.

Contents

Introduction

In Greek mythology, a king called Sisyphus was cursed for his past excesses. His solitary punishment was to push an immense boulder up a steep hill, only to have it roll back down and the task to start all over again. Diabetes might also seem like a curse to an eternity of useless repetition and unending frustration, but it's not like that at all.

First, your goals of understanding and managing your diabetes are achievable. With the application of good diabetes care, healthy nutrition and regular physical activity, most people with type 2 diabetes lead full and healthy lives. Your effort is never futile.

Second, managing diabetes is not as hard as it sounds. What might appear on the surface to be an enormous or complex undertaking can become quite effortless with practice and application.

Third, diabetes management is not a punishment. It is easy to fall into the trap of believing that some suffering is the price of good health, like the distasteful medicine you must swallow to get well. But dieting is not punishment for the nutritionally wicked, nor is exercise the castigation of the couch potato. These are positive steps that have their own rewards.

Fourth, diabetes management requires a careful coordination of physical activity, diet and medication. But this does not mean you have to do the same things every day or eat the same restrictive diet, trapped in a tedious and repetitive cycle of care. In fact, diabetes management can be very flexible, matching individual requirements and capabilities with diet, exercise or medications.

Finally, you are not alone with your burden. Diabetes management will harness the support of your doctor, diabetes

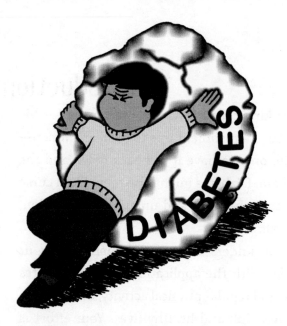

Diabetes can sometimes feel like a curse to a lifetime of futile repetition. But it is not like this at all!

educator, dietician, podiatrist and many other professionals that comprise your diabetes care team. Each person will help you manage your diabetes and make the task of managing diabetes not only feasible but also revitalising.

This book is your guide to diabetes and outlines the many opportunities you have to make a positive difference to your health. It begins by examining what diabetes is and how it comes about. It then goes on to describe the many practical changes you can make to your diet, and the potential strengths as well as weaknesses of these changes. It also looks at physical activity and the different ways exercise can be used to both maintain and improve your health. The book also explores the medical aspects of diabetes care, including practical ways to achieve control of your waistline, blood glucose, blood pressure and cholesterol levels, as well as the best means to avoid major complications.

You can do this. It is nothing like pushing a rock up a hill.

1.
What is diabetes?

UNDERSTAND

» The human body runs on fuel, like the petrol in your car. Glucose is chiefly used to fuel chemical reactions inside the body.

» To keep the brain and body healthy, blood glucose levels are normally kept within a narrow range, balanced by the actions of insulin and other hormones.

» Insulin is made and released by the beta-cells of the pancreas to coordinate the body's response to rising glucose levels.

» Diabetes occurs when there is not enough insulin (function) to keep glucose levels under control.

» High glucose levels usually start out as a silent problem. Most people diagnosed with type 2 diabetes are completely unaware they have it, and have probably had it for many years.

MANAGE

» Recognise what your own symptoms of high glucose levels are and how they might be affecting your health and wellbeing.

» Frequently assess how well your glucose levels are being controlled with the help of your diabetes care team.

» Work with your diabetes care team to define the most appropriate targets for the intensity of your own glucose control.

» Learn to monitor your own glucose levels using a blood glucose meter.

» Follow and learn what different foods or activities do to your glucose levels, and use this information to develop diet and lifestyle plans that best meet your individual needs.

The name **glucose** comes from the Greek word *glukus*, meaning 'sweet'. Glucose is a simple sugar. Because glucose is the major sugar inside the human body, the terms 'glucose' and 'sugar' are often used interchangeably when managing diabetes. But glucose is not the same thing as the white sugar used in cooking or in your coffee.

The human body runs on fuel, like the petrol in your car. Glucose is chiefly used to fuel chemical reactions inside the body. This is known as **metabolism**. Metabolism provides the vital energy for every cell to do what needs to be done. For your brain's metabolism, glucose is absolutely essential. Yet the brain has little stored glucose of its own and no other fuel to burn if glucose runs out. Instead, it relies on the glucose dissolved in the blood to maintain continuous supply and continuous functioning. From the brain's point of view, blood glucose is as important as the oxygen in the air you breathe: it can only function for a few minutes without either before it stops working altogether.

To guarantee your brain keeps running night and day, the body must ensure that glucose is always present in your blood in roughly the same concentration. To achieve this level of control is not easy. Some days you might eat a few pieces of chocolate cake or a bowl of spaghetti. Other times you might eat hardly anything at all. Yet through it all, glucose levels will normally fluctuate only very slightly:

» between 4–6mmol/L (72–108mg/dL) when not eating and
» between 4–7mmol/L (72–126mg/dL) after a meal.

This amazing level of control is achieved thanks to an elaborate system of checks and balances that carefully regulates how much glucose is going into the blood and how much is going out.

In essence, diabetes is the state in which this balance fails and glucose levels rise.

Every time you eat or drink something that contains any **carbohydrate** (also known as **carbs**) your body gets a dose of glucose. Whether you are eating chocolate cake or spaghetti or drinking a Coke, the carbs contained in each product are broken down by your digestion into simple sugars, one of which is glucose. As these sugars are digested and absorbed, they trigger the release of hormones, the most important of which is **insulin**. Hormones are chemical signals that communicate a message from one part of the body to another, usually via the bloodstream. Insulin is made and released by the **beta-cells of the pancreas**. The message insulin sends coordinates the body's response to rising blood glucose levels. This message tells the cells of the liver, muscles and fat to take away glucose from the blood (and store it for later use). It also tells the liver to stop making and releasing any extra glucose, which is rendered unnecessary by having just had a meal.

This is a proportional response. The greater the amount of glucose contained in a product and the faster it hits your system, the greater the amount of insulin that is released. This keeps glucose levels from rising too fast or too high. In contrast, a meal that is low in sugar or contains sugars that are only slowly digested will need to trigger a proportionally smaller insulin response to make sure glucose levels don't drop too rapidly.

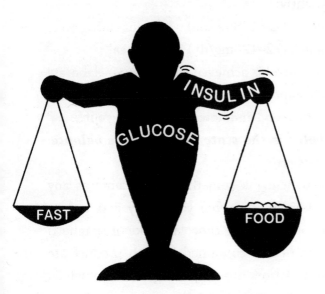

Diabetes occurs when there is not enough insulin (function) to keep glucose levels balanced.

The net result of this finely balanced system is that, in people without diabetes, glucose levels in the blood only rise slightly and very briefly following a meal, regardless of what they eat.

When you are not eating, your brain still needs glucose to keep functioning. So to keep up with the brain's unceasing demands, the liver slowly releases its glucose stores and also manufactures new glucose, which it releases into the blood in a kind of controlled drip feed for the brain. To make this happen as soon as glucose levels start to fall, the pancreas immediately stops releasing insulin and starts making other hormones such as **glucagon**. These hormones send a different message. They now say that any unnecessary uptake of glucose must stop and the brakes that insulin has placed on the liver's glucose production should be removed. Again, the rate at which glucose is released into the blood is finely balanced to match the rate at which the body (and in particular the brain) uses glucose. So glucose levels in the blood don't fall very much, if at all, between meals in people who do not have diabetes. Even if they skip a meal, or wish to fast for several days, glucose levels always remain sufficient for the brain to keep working.

So in people without diabetes, day and night, feeding or fasting, the levels of glucose in their blood do not rise or fall much at all, balanced by the actions of insulin and other hormones.

Diabetes occurs when there is not enough insulin (function) to keep glucose levels under control.

How and why this happens is complicated. Many different factors can contribute to the decline and loss of insulin's functions, leading ultimately to the development of type 2 diabetes. These are discussed in detail in Chapter 2.

Diabetes and glucose control

Not having enough insulin has two major consequences for glucose control.

1. In diabetes, glucose levels rise in the blood after a meal

As the job of insulin is chiefly to coordinate your body to deal with the sugars in your meal, one of the first signs that insulin is not doing this job is a rise in your glucose level after a meal, especially after a big carbohydrate-rich meal. This is when you need to make the greatest amount of insulin to cope with the extra glucose entering your blood, so this is also when any limited capacity for insulin production is first challenged.

One simple way to test for type 2 diabetes is an **oral glucose tolerance test** (**OGTT**). This test involves drinking a large amount of glucose and then determining how quickly it is cleared from the blood and glucose balance is restored. It is essentially a 'road test' of your pancreas to see if it can rev up and handle the (sugar) hills. An OGTT is usually performed in the morning after having not eaten anything overnight. Drinking water beforehand is allowed, but no coffee, tea or juice. At the start of the OGTT a blood sample is drawn. You are then given a sweet solution (containing 75g of glucose) to drink within 5 minutes. A further blood sample is drawn 2 hours later and the glucose level is measured.

In healthy people, the glucose level in their blood 2 hours after drinking the glucose will be below 7.8mmol/L (140mg/dL). If your glucose level is above 11mmol/L (198mg/dL) 2 hours after drinking the glucose, this indicates a diagnosis of diabetes. If glucose levels are modestly elevated (between 7.8 and 11mmol/L) (140.4 and 198mg/dL) then **impaired glucose tolerance** is said to exist. This is also known as **pre-diabetes**, as without significant changes in diet and lifestyle many people with these intermediate levels ultimately go on to develop full-blown diabetes.

2. In diabetes, glucose levels stay up even when you are not eating

Most of the glucose in your blood has not come from your diet. It has been made and released by your liver. As detailed earlier in this chapter, in the healthy human body the production of glucose is perfectly in tune with the glucose levels in your blood and the rate at which it is used up. So glucose levels in the blood do not fall very much when you are not eating.

If glucose levels are too high, unnecessary glucose production by the liver should be shut down, so balancing the system. But in type 2 diabetes this does not happen very well. This is partly because there is not enough insulin (function) to stop glucose production. In addition, the signals that drive glucose production, like glucagon and free fat in the blood, fail to be adequately suppressed.

In essence, your liver mistakenly believes you are hungry and need more glucose, even when you have just eaten.

So in diabetes too much glucose is made by the liver and released into your blood, especially considering that glucose levels are already high. Consequently, glucose levels can remain elevated in people with type 2 diabetes even if they are on a stringent diet or are eating almost nothing at all. Indeed, most people are first diagnosed with type 2 diabetes because they are found to have a glucose level greater than 7mmol/L (126 mg/dL) on a routine blood test taken when they were not eating (e.g. before a meal).

For the same reasons, avoiding all pleasurable sugary foods and drinks, which has been the mainstay of diabetes management for many years, makes less sense if most glucose is coming from your liver. In fact, most people with diabetes can eat the same amount of dessert and other sweet foods as people without diabetes, without ever compromising their glucose control (see Chapter 3).

The consequences of high glucose levels

High glucose levels usually start out as a silent problem. Many people are completely unaware they have type 2 diabetes. Yet glucose levels have usually been elevated in the blood for an average of 5 to 10 years before a diagnosis of type 2 diabetes is first made.

The most common symptoms associated with type 2 diabetes are easily dismissed as a signs of getting old or other problems. These may include:

» feeling tired and weak all the time
» having difficulty concentrating
» feeling restless and uncomfortable
» not doing the things you usually do with the same skill or enthusiasm
» finding the things that were difficult now even harder to do
» trouble with your eyesight and/or dry eyes
» dry and itchy skin
» yeast infections in the feet, groin and under your breasts
» being irritable or moody
» reduced interest in (and difficulties during) sex
» general aches and pains
» passing urine more frequently during the day and especially during the night
» feeling thirsty and hungry, even though you seem to be drinking and eating more
» difficulty getting to sleep and staying asleep and/or waking up still feeling 'hung over'.

There is nothing here that is unique to type 2 diabetes. So looking for diabetes as the cause of these symptoms usually takes a modicum of suspicion. Once diagnosed, however, it is usually obvious that type 2 diabetes has been making your life miserable for some time.

All of these symptoms are caused by having high glucose levels in your blood. They are not permanent or a sign of damage. When diabetes is treated and glucose control is restored most of these symptoms will go away. This is one reason why you and your diabetes care team will be working to keep your glucose levels as close to normal as possible.

The other important reason for wanting to regain control of your glucose levels is that, in the long term, high glucose levels can be toxic to many parts of the body, especially the blood vessels, heart, nerves, eyes, bladder and kidneys. This can result in serious and life-threatening damage in some people with type 2 diabetes, but certainly not in everyone. These so-called **complications of diabetes** are not an inevitable result of high glucose levels. They are definitely more common in those people who struggle to keep control of their glucose levels. However, glucose control is not enough on its own to completely keep these complications at bay. A comprehensive approach to the most important complications of diabetes is presented in detail in the latter half of this book.

Glucose monitoring using HbA1c

The most common way to get a handle on your glucose control is for a doctor to measure your **haemoglobin A1c** (also known as **HbA1c** or **A1c**). The test for this involves having a blood sample taken and sent away to a clinical laboratory. The HbA1c shows the amount of glucose that is stuck onto to a protein — haemoglobin — in your red blood cells. The higher your glucose levels have been during the previous 3 to 4 months, the more glucose will be stuck to the haemoglobin and the higher your HbA1c will be. But if you have been able to improve your glucose control over this time period, your HbA1c will fall.

In people without diabetes, their HbA1c is almost always less than 6 per cent (or 48mmol/mol in the new units for this test now used by many doctors). By comparison, without treatment, people with type 2 diabetes usually have an HbA1c of greater than 6.5 per cent (50mmol/mol). This means that taking a blood test to measure your HbA1c can also be used to confirm if you have diabetes.

An HbA1c greater than 8 per cent (64mmol/mol) suggests

persistently elevated glucose levels and generally indicates the blood glucose is not well controlled and the risk of complications is increased.

Your HbA1c will be measured when you are diagnosed with type 2 diabetes and then at least twice a year thereafter. It is also common to measure your HbA1c about 3 months after starting any new treatment to lower your glucose levels, as it takes this long for its full effect to be seen on your HbA1c.

Often the first step in diabetes management will be to set an appropriate target for your HbA1c that takes into account your age, lifestyle, work practices, the treatment you are receiving and a host of other factors. Ideally, the aim of diabetes management is to keep glucose levels as close as possible to those found in people without diabetes. But in practical terms, getting and keeping the HbA1c to less than 7 per cent (or 53mmol/mol) is as good as it gets in diabetes. And this is probably all that's necessary. This degree of control will eliminate most of the symptoms caused by high glucose levels. In addition, improving glucose control beyond this does not appreciably reduce your risk of complications, while potentially exposing you to more side effects from your medications (see Chapter 5). However, sometimes even aiming for this level of glucose control is not the right thing for you to do. This kind of individualised assessment of your current level of glucose control, and the value and safety of going lower, will be made almost every time you see your doctor.

Monitoring using blood glucose levels

Another way to come to grips with your glucose control is to directly measure and monitor your own blood glucose levels using a **blood glucose meter**. This is known as **self-monitoring**. The glucose test involves pricking your finger to release a drop of blood. It is not very painful or particularly complicated to do. The drop of blood is then applied to a plastic strip and placed in a small machine that measures the glucose level in the blood.

When glucose levels are under good control, most of the results from self-monitoring will be between:

»   6–8mmol/L (108–144mg/dL) when not eating and before meals, and

»   6–10mmol/L (108–180mg/dL) after a meal.

Testing your own blood glucose levels is a practical way to make sure yourself that your diabetes management is on track. Self-monitoring also enables you to find out how different foods and activities affect your own individual blood glucose levels, and makes it easier to develop and modify diet and lifestyle plans that best suit your individual needs. In addition, self-monitoring provides valuable and prompt feedback about anything you might be doing to improve your glucose control, such as changes in your medication, physical activity, diet or lifestyle. Blood glucose monitoring can also be a useful way to reduce the risk of hypoglycaemia (see Chapter 5).

It is not essential to monitor your own glucose levels. However, most people with type 2 diabetes are encouraged to when there is adequate training, support and assessment.

A strategic plan for blood glucose monitoring will usually be developed in conjunction with your diabetes care team. The frequency of self-monitoring will always need to be different for different people and different situations. For example, people with very stable control may need to monitor less often than those starting out on a new treatment regimen, or those troubled by lots of highs and/or lows. How often you need to test may range from once or twice a week to many times a day, timed to coincide with key problem periods. More testing will usually be undertaken if you are unwell, because this is commonly the time that glucose control, as well as other aspects of your health, goes awry.

A new way to monitor glucose levels has recently become more widely available. This is known as **continuous glucose monitoring (CGM)** and involves wearing a small device that is able to measure glucose levels every 5 minutes. It can be worn for up to 6 days and can track changes in your glucose levels throughout the day and night. Some devices also have alarms for glucose highs and lows. These devices can provide a very accurate picture of your daily fluctuations in blood glucose control and help find the best approach to tackling your own individual glucose control problems. At present, CGM devices are mostly used only for brief periods, and give a brief snapshot of glucose control over a few days. However, some people are starting to use this technology every day. It is likely that the future management of diabetes will increasingly involve continuous blood glucose monitoring.

2

Why did it happen to me?

UNDERSTAND

» Many different factors can contribute to the decline and loss of insulin's functions, leading ultimately to the development of type 2 diabetes.

» By the time type 2 diabetes is diagnosed it may be that over half of the insulin-producing beta-cells in the pancreas have been lost.

» Beta-cells may become progressively exhausted because of the demands of an unhealthy diet or having to work against insulin resistance to keep your metabolism under control.

» Most people develop type 2 diabetes because they cannot safely contain the excess energy from their diet and a 'toxic waist' starts to accumulate.

» To develop type 2 diabetes, you also need to be susceptible either to developing ectopic fat or your beta-cells must be susceptible to exhaustion, which can be the result of genes, ethnicity or acquired during your development or as you age.

MANAGE

» Unburden your pancreas from too much work by reducing the carbs and calories you eat, and slowing their delivery using low GI, high fibre substitutes.

» Measure your waist circumference and compare it to what it should be in someone of your gender and ethnic background. Set targets to make it smaller.

» Increase your level of physical activity to achieve a negative energy balance that will help to remove ectopic fat from your body.

» Restrict the amount of energy you get from your food and drink by improving your dietary choices or adhering to a diet.

Diabetes is a simple disease. It occurs when there is not enough insulin (function) to keep your glucose levels under control. Insulin is a hormone made and released by the beta-cells of the pancreas. Its job is to coordinate the body's response to rising blood glucose levels in the blood. Diabetes develops only when it can't do this anymore. But while diabetes is a simple problem, the reasons why diabetes comes about are much more complex. *Many different factors can contribute to the decline and loss of insulin's functions, leading ultimately to the development of diabetes.*

In some people, the immune system can inadvertently destroy the insulin-producing beta-cells of the pancreas. This is called **type 1 diabetes**. Type 1 diabetes accounts for around 8 to 10 per cent of all people with diabetes. It can occur at any age, not just in children and adolescents. Type 1 diabetes used to be known as **insulin-dependent diabetes** because the ability to make insulin is completely lost and insulin injections are always needed to survive. However, people with other forms of diabetes may also need insulin to control their glucose levels, so this name has become obsolete.

The most common form of diabetes is **type 2 diabetes**, which accounts for over 90 per cent of all diabetes in adults.

In type 2 diabetes, the capacity to produce enough insulin to adequately control your glucose levels is progressively exhausted over many years (probably at least 20 years). By the time type 2 diabetes is finally diagnosed it may be that over half of the insulin-producing beta-cells in the pancreas have been lost.

What causes type 2 diabetes?

Broadly, there are three inter-related factors that hurt the beta-cells of the pancreas. These act to a greater or lesser extent in different people, but cumulatively they mean that the capacity for insulin production eventually fails to keep up with demands, and glucose levels start to rise.

Too much work can be exhausting

The beta-cells of the pancreas normally make insulin in proportion to the amount of glucose in a meal and how quickly it is digested and absorbed (known as the **glycaemic load** or **GL** — see Chapter 3). If you subject your pancreas to a diet rich in sugars, especially those that are readily digested, your pancreas will have to make more insulin. And these excessive demands to make more and more insulin eventually take their toll. Certainly, people who habitually eat this kind of unhealthy diet also have a higher risk of developing type 2 diabetes.

The pancreas will also have to work harder if the cells of the body become less sensitive to insulin (known as insulin resistance).

To compensate, much more insulin must be made and released to keep glucose under control. This is like driving with the handbrake still partly on — it takes more revs to get anywhere and eventually damages your engine.

Another time when insulin resistance can become a problem

is during pregnancy. In every pregnancy, hormones and other factors normally cause resistance to the actions of insulin. This means that insulin production in pregnant women needs to be almost doubled to keep glucose levels under control. Most women's bodies can do this. However, some women do not have the capacity to double their insulin production, especially older and/or overweight women. And again, when there is not enough insulin (function) to keep metabolism under control, glucose levels rise and diabetes occurs. When this happens during pregnancy it is known as **gestational diabetes**. Although glucose levels usually return to normal after giving birth, women with gestational diabetes are four times more likely to develop type 2 diabetes as they age when compared to those who have a diabetes-free pregnancy. Many people think of a 9-month pregnancy as a kind of road test for what might happen in the future should you remain overweight or inactive over much longer periods as, like pregnancy, all of these things cause a degree of resistance to the effects of insulin and require your pancreas to work much harder.

Another condition associated with type 2 diabetes is **polycystic ovarian syndrome** (or **PCOS**). PCOS affects between 5 to 10 per cent of all women. It can cause women to experience irregular periods, acne, and excessive facial hair and weight gain. Having PCOS also makes you more likely to develop type 2 diabetes, which may affect up to 40 per cent of women with PCOS by the time they are 40 years old. This is partly because those women with PCOS also have great resistance to the (glucose-lowering) actions of insulin.

Some medicines used in the treatment of other diseases may also cause type 2 diabetes in some people through making the body more resistant to the effects of insulin. These include steroid pills (especially in high doses), some diuretics and antipsychotics used in the treatment of mental illness.

Too much fat in all the wrong places

Most people develop type 2 diabetes because they cannot safely contain the excess energy from their diet and a **toxic waist** starts to accumulate.

Most of the excess energy from your diet is stored as fat. The equation is simple: if you eat it and you don't burn it in your metabolism or physical activities, then you store it. Energy is too precious a thing for the body to waste.

Your fat normally turns over about 10 per cent of its energy stores every day. This means it always has plenty in reserve in case of extra requirements, such as if you miss a meal or need to be more active than usual.

The body initially stores its fat mostly under the skin, in the thighs, buttocks and breasts (known as **peripheral fat**). These depots are very efficient at impounding fat and keeping it safe until its energy is needed. This is partly because peripheral fat is sensitive to the signals that regulate metabolism, the most important of which is **insulin**, which promotes fat storage.

Peripheral fat is not unhealthy. If you remove all this fat from under your skin (by liposuction) you do not become any healthier or reduce your chances of developing type 2 diabetes. In fact, it is thought that having this kind of healthy fat might prevent the dangerous spill-over of fat into other tissues. Transplanting peripheral fat into people who have an abnormal deficiency of fat tissue (known as lipodystrophy) can actually improve their health.

The problem comes when these peripheral fat stores are filled up or stop listening to insulin. If they can no longer act as an energy reservoir, what do you do with all the extra energy now? You can't afford to waste it. So you need to build additional storage capacity outside of where fat is normally stored. This is known as **ectopic fat**. Most of these new 'dump sites' are around the internal organs (also known as **visceral fat**) or inside them (known as **steatosis**).

The easiest way to determine whether you have any of this ectopic fat is to place a tape measure around your waist, two finger breadths above the top of your hip bone.

A healthy waist circumference is considered to be
» **for men: less than 94cm (37in) (Asian men: less than 90cm/35½in)**
» **for women: less than 80cm (31½in) (Asian women: less than 80cm/31½in).**

Few people with a waist circumference persistently in the healthy reference range will ever develop type 2 diabetes. By contrast, over 90 per cent of people with type 2 diabetes will have been much rounder than this when their diabetes was first identified. As your waistline increases beyond these levels, the chances that you might develop type 2 diabetes will significantly increase. Diabetes is not inevitable if you are overweight, but it does become more likely. For example, when compared to people with a healthy waist circumference, developing diabetes in the next 5 years is four times more likely if you have a waistline that is:
» greater than 102cm (40in) in men (Asian men: greater than 90cm/35½in)
» greater than 88cm (34½in) women (Asian women: greater than 80cm/31½in).
At least three out of four people with type 2 diabetes have a waist circumference in this range (known as **abdominal obesity**).

Most people develop type 2 diabetes because they cannot safely store the excess energy from their diet and a 'toxic waist' starts to accumulate.

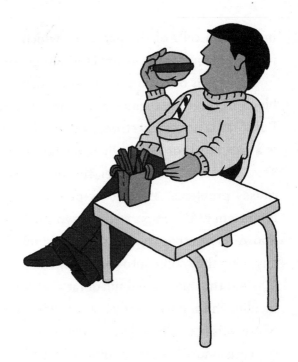

This implies that they also have a large amount of ectopic fat in their body. In fact, if you directly look for an excess of (ectopic) fat in the liver (known as **fatty liver** or **hepatic steatosis**) you find that at least three out of four people with type 2 diabetes also have too much fat here too.

The problem with ectopic fat is that it is not very good at its job. It is really a makeshift solution to the 'problem of fat storage'. The French term is *pis aller* (*pis* = worse; *aller* = to go; literally 'the worst going'). And in not doing its job very well, a number of things can go wrong. In particular, ectopic fat is far less efficient at safekeeping its fat stores. It tries really hard to compensate and is much more metabolically active than peripheral fat, but it is just not very good at it. Instead, fat leaches out into the tissues and the blood, particularly after a meal, when levels should normally be going down. These free fats and their by-products are directly toxic in many parts of the body, including in the beta-cells of the pancreas, which accumulate ectopic fat in great globules that ultimately change the way they function.

Free fat is only supposed to be a drip feed, released into the blood in carefully regulated amounts when you are not eating. But if fat is not safely stored, and levels are high in the blood, it is a free meal for cells, which get fatter themselves as a result. This excessive flux of fuel through a cell's metabolism also causes problems, as toxic by-products are generated through inefficiency. The most well known are the **free radicals** (also known as reactive oxygen species), which react with and damage anything they come into contact with.

Cells that are stuffed full of fat also don't respond that well to insulin. This is particularly the case when ectopic fat accumulates in the cells of the liver. As detailed above, this forces the pancreas to overproduce insulin to compensate for insulin resistance. And this means more work for the beta-cells of the pancreas, which are already feeling the strain.

Finally, fat is not a lifeless lump of lard. In fact, it is a dynamic regulator of health and wellbeing. All fat, but especially ectopic fat, is able to produce a range of chemicals that affect metabolism, inflammation, blood pressure and many other functions (known as **adipokines**). In fact, fat tissue is the largest producer of hormones in the human body. People with type 2 diabetes often have high levels of adipokines. Some of these adipokines can oppose the function of insulin and cause insulin resistance.

You also need to be susceptible

There are a great many people who are overweight, some of them extremely so. But only a minority develop type 2 diabetes. This is because you also need a third factor to be present for type 2 diabetes to occur.

To develop type 2 diabetes, you also need to be susceptible either to developing ectopic fat or your beta-cells must be susceptible to exhaustion.

Some people are better than others at safely setting aside any excess energy from their diet as healthy peripheral fat. This might be because they have a bigger storage capacity or are more able to expand it when needed, rather than dumping fat around their organs. What determines when the peripheral fat store reaches its capacity (in essence its size and expandability) may be different in different people depending on their age, gender, race, genes and a host of other factors.

For example, people of Asian descent are generally more prone to lay down fat around their organs if they eat too much or are inactive. This is because Asian people have a leaner build with a lower storage capacity in their peripheral fat. Consequently, if you are Asian, gaining 5kg (11lb) in weight almost doubles your risk of type 2 diabetes. By comparison a 5kg (11lb) weight gain in a Caucasian person has less than half this effect.

Diabetes also doesn't affect everyone who has resistance to the effects of insulin or everyone who is eating a bad diet. This appears to be because some people remain quite capable of making enough insulin to control their glucose levels even though they may need to make very large amounts of insulin in the face of stiff insulin resistance or dietary excesses. However, other people simply can't sustain this extra workload for long and eventually there is not enough insulin (function) to keep glucose levels under control, and type 2 diabetes develops.

There may be a number of different factors that make your pancreas susceptible to the effects of too much work or too much fat.

In the family

Type 2 diabetes tends to run in families. One in every three people with type 2 diabetes also has a close family member with type 2 diabetes. If either of your parents, your brother or your sister has type 2 diabetes, you are five to six times more likely to develop type 2 diabetes yourself. If three family members have type 2 diabetes, you are over fifteen times more likely to develop type 2 diabetes yourself than someone without a family history. The reason that type 2 diabetes runs in families is partly due to similar diet, lifestyle habits and exposure to environmental factors. It may also be partly determined by your genes.

Genes are the basic instructions encoded in your DNA that are used to determine how your body works. These gene instructions are passed down from parents to their children, who all share similar genes. In some cases, the genes you inherit may increase your risk of type 2 diabetes. Most of these genes appear to influence how well beta-cells handle the stress of having to make more insulin. But while genes are important in some families, overall they explain only a small fraction of why most people develop type 2 diabetes.

During early development

Susceptibility to type 2 diabetes may also be acquired during your life, particularly during your early development in your mother's womb. For example, babies very small for their age have an increased risk of developing type 2 diabetes when they grow up. This is probably because the same thing that restricts the growth of a baby also restricts the development of the pancreas and ultimately its capacity to take the strain of controlling glucose levels during adulthood. A mother's high glucose levels during pregnancy can also increase the risk of type 2 diabetes in her children, partly because their beta-cells become more susceptible to damage.

Increased susceptibility with ageing

Some people develop type 2 diabetes only when they are very old, without having been very overweight or inactive during their life. This is probably because the regenerative capacity of the pancreas is not limitless, and the ability to make insulin slowly declines with time in everyone. But ageing just brings you closer to the edge — usually something else is also required to push you over. Whether 'getting old' will result in type 2 diabetes is determined by how great the demands are for insulin production and how great this capacity has already been reduced by other factors. Of those people who develop type 2 diabetes in their eighties, it is often suggested that it was probably always going to happen no matter what, given enough time. But if these same people had been overweight and inactive during their lives, it would probably have happened much earlier.

Type 2 diabetes: three strikes and you're out

Type 2 diabetes will affect at least one in every three people at some point during their lifetime. But it will not affect everyone.

There are many people who are overweight who don't get diabetes. There are many who have a poor diet or the wrong genes, and they don't get diabetes either. To get type 2 diabetes you need all three things to happen.

» You need the beta-cells of the pancreas to be overworked.
» You need too much fat in the wrong places.
» You need to be susceptible (such that your ability to compensate for overwork of your beta-cells and too much fat in your body ultimately fails).

Type 2 diabetes is made more likely if any one of these factors is increased. For example, an unhealthy diet will increase the work of the pancreas and increase the risk of diabetes. Similarly, being overweight can increase your risk of diabetes even without a strong family history. Equally, some people have a strong family history of diabetes so it doesn't take much extra work or being very overweight for diabetes to occur. Of course, if more than one of these factors is increased, your risk will multiply and diabetes will become both more likely and more likely to occur at an earlier age.

At the same time, the best ways to prevent and treat diabetes will target these important areas. For example, changes in the amount and types of sugar and fibre in your diet can reduce the strain on your pancreas to produce large amounts of insulin (see Chapter 3). Getting rid of any extra fat in your body through diet (Chapter 4) and increased physical activity (Chapter 5) will reduce its limiting effects on your metabolism. Some medicines will also help to protect the beta-cells and make them more able to compensate for the demands of glucose control.

In its early stages, diabetes is potentially reversible. Gastric bypass surgery dramatically reduces food intake and causes a great decline in the amount of ectopic fat in your body (see Chapter 4). This is able to 'cure' type 2 diabetes such that many people having this procedure can keep control of their glucose levels without the need for any medications. While it requires complicated, invasive major surgery that is not suitable for most people with type 2 diabetes, it does illustrate that once you understand the factors involved in the development of diabetes, and target them aggressively, anything is possible.

3

A spoon less of sugar

UNDERSTAND

» Reducing the demands on your pancreas to make insulin can be achieved by reducing the amount of carbohydrates you eat and/or changing the type of carbohydrates you eat.

» You can reduce the amount of carbs you eat by following a diet or meal plan that is low in carbs (low carb diet) or by restricting the amount of carbs you eat through carb counting.

» Sugar substitutes and sweeteners can safely reduce the carbs in your diet, as between 10 and 15 per cent of the energy in carbs probably comes from added sugars.

» Some foods have greater and faster effects on your glucose control than others. This can be estimated as their glycaemic index or GI.

» Dietary fibre plays an important role in good glucose control, even though it is not digested by your body.

MANAGE

» Incorporate a serve of fruit and vegetables into every meal.

» Explore the nutritional information guide on the foods you currently eat, or download a program for your phone to help you do this on the fly. Look at the content of carbs, fibre and GI where available.

» Experiment with different recipes that use sugar substitutes and find a product that works for your tastebuds as well as your glucose control.

» Find new ways to put fibre into your diet by substituting wholegrain alternatives, bran or fruit, or using fibre supplements.

» Monitor your glucose control, as improvements that come from changes in the amount or type of carbohydrate in your diet can reduce your requirements for certain glucose-lowering medications.

A hundred years ago, the only rational treatment for type 2 diabetes was to avoid all carbohydrate in your diet. It is still widely thought that having type 2 diabetes only means you have to avoid sugar and any sweet foods and drinks that contain it. While this is not strictly true, managing your carbohydrate intake is one important strategy for achieving and maintaining good glucose control.

Almost all food contains some **carbohydrate** (also known as **carbs**). Some of the carbohydrate in your diet is in the form of simple sugars, like sucrose (the white 'table sugar') and fructose (in fruit and honey). Your tastebuds are able to detect the presence of simple sugars in food or drink, which is why such things taste sweet. Simple sugars occur naturally in sweet foods or may be added in food processing or by consumers (e.g. into your coffee) for extra sweetness. On average, between 10 and 15 per cent of the total energy (calories) in your diet comes from these added sugars, but in some people's diets this can exceed 25 per cent.

However, most carbohydrate in your diet is in the form of complex chains of hundreds to thousands of glucose molecules.

This is known as **starch**. Starch is the major store of energy in plants and is found in many plant-based foods, from bread and cereal to pasta and rice. It does not taste sweet as its sugars are locked up into these complex chains. However, starch is rapidly digested in your intestines, where its sugars are released and subsequently absorbed into the bloodstream in precisely the same way as table sugar.

As any sugar is digested and absorbed, it triggers the release of hormones. The most important of these is **insulin**, which coordinates the body's response to ensure the levels of glucose in your blood rise only slightly after a meal, if at all. This is a proportionate response: the greater the amount of carbohydrate in a meal and the faster it is digested and absorbed, the more insulin that needs to be made to keep your glucose levels from rising dangerously. The combined effects of these two components — the quantity and quality of carbohydrate in a meal — is known as the **glycaemic load (GL)**. Essentially, GL is an estimate of the demand placed on your pancreas to make insulin by any particular meal.

Of course, what happens in type 2 diabetes is that there is not always enough insulin to keep glucose under control, especially after meals.

So one way to make sure that your limited capacity for insulin production will still be enough to keep control is to reduce the glycaemic load imparted by your diet.

This can be done in essentially two different ways:

» by reducing the amount of carbs you eat (e.g. following a low carb diet, carb counting or using sugar substitutes)
» by slowing the absorption of carbs from your diet by carefully selecting the carbs you eat (by their GI index) and/ or by substituting more soluble fibre into your meals.

This chapter will look in detail at these two common ways to manage diabetes and their role in helping to improve your glucose control. Although discussed separately, there is no reason why some or all of these interventions can't be combined for even better glucose control. In addition, changes in your diet have a far greater role in managing diabetes than just making your glucose levels easier to control. A good diet will improve waist management, the control of lipids and blood pressure levels as well as the prevention of complications. These facets are discussed in specific chapters dedicated to these topics found elsewhere in this book. This chapter will just look at how it is possible to reduce the rise in glucose levels after a meal by making changes to your diet.

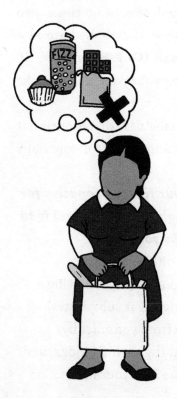

One way to make sure your limited capacity to produce insulin is still enough to keep glucose under control is to slow the absorption of sugars from your diet.

Low carbohydrate diets

Low carb diets have become very popular for the management of type 2 diabetes. In theory, by reducing the amount or proportion of carbohydrate you are eating you can also reduce the demands on your pancreas to make insulin. So if you have only a limited capacity to make insulin, as occurs in people with type 2 diabetes, reducing the carbohydrate component in your diet can make it more likely your limited capacity will be sufficient to keep control of your glucose levels.

Typically, half of the energy in a standard diet comes from carbohydrates. In fact, because of the push from modern consumers to reduce the amount of fat in their diets, people in the 21st century are eating more carbohydrates than ever before. Diabetes may be one of the consequences.

Carbohydrates are found in high proportions in many common foods, including:

» breads, biscuits/cookies and cereals
» pasta, rice, noodles and grains (such as oats and barley)
» starchy vegetables such as potatoes, corn and peas
» milk and yoghurt
» fruits and juices.

In low carb diets, any foods that are high in carbohydrates are strictly limited or substituted with foods containing more proteins and/or more fats (e.g. meat, poultry, fish, shellfish, eggs, cheese, nuts and seeds). Alternatively, some low carb diets simply replace common carb-rich products with other foods that are essentially low in carbohydrates (e.g. non-starchy salad vegetables for potatoes or rice). Generally, low carb diets mean you eat differently rather than eating less.

Perhaps the most well-known example of a low carb diet is the Atkins Diet. However, there are a range of other diets that share roughly the same principles with respect to carbs but vary in their relative amounts of other nutrients (e.g. how much fat or protein you eat).

Carb counting

Limiting your carbohydrate intake is relatively easy to achieve by yourself, simply by estimating how many carbs are contained in different products then planning your meal and how much of it you will eat to match your chosen limit. This practice is known as **carbohydrate counting** or **counting carbs** and is widely recommended for people with type 2 diabetes as a means to control their blood glucose levels.

Some information about the carbs in your food can be obtained simply by reading the 'nutritional information panel' present on the labels of most processed foods. Look first at the **serving size** section. All the information below it will be about what you will get when you eat this amount of this product. If you eat more than this, which is usually the case with most of these products, all the nutrients you will be getting will increase proportionally, including the carbs.

On the label, total carbohydrates are measured in grams (g), for instance, one serve is said to be equal to 15g of carbohydrate. When counting carbs it is common to subtract half the amount of fibre from the total amount of carbohydrate to determine what is known as the **effective carbs** or **net carbs**. For example, if a product contains 23g of carbohydrate (total) and 6g of fibre, then its net carbs will be around 20g per serve. This figure approximates the amount of carbohydrate in a product that will impact on insulin production and potentially your blood glucose levels. It is also another good reason to choose high fibre products which have their own benefits (detailed below).

Most of the food we commonly eat has no labels at all. There is approximately 15g of net carbohydrate in:

» one slice of bread
» 1 tablespoon of syrup, jam, jelly, sugar or honey
» one piece of fresh fruit
» ⅔ cup of plain fat-free yoghurt or yoghurt sweetened with sugar substitute
» two to three biscuits/cookies
» ⅓ muffin
» ⅓ cup of pasta or rice
» ⅓ of a large baked potato.

There are also many recipe books, websites and phone apps now available that provide useful information about how many carbs are contained in most kinds of food and drinks, which can help in planning your meals.

A typical low carb diet will aim to limit carbs to only five to ten serves a day. A good place to start is to limit your carbohydrate intake to no more than three to four serves (45–60g) of carbs in each meal, or no more than ten serves (150g) of carbs each day.

The maths involved in calculating carbs is not as hard as it sounds and becomes easier as you go. Often a dietician will get you started with meal plans based on fixed serves of carbohydrate spread throughout the day. This also makes it easier to control your glucose levels after meals, as when you know what's coming you also know what it will do to your glucose levels.

Low carb and type 2 diabetes

A number of studies have consistently shown that low carb diets and carb counting are able to improve glucose control in people with type 2 diabetes. This may be partly because these strategies can also cause weight loss, which is often achieved quite rapidly much to the delight of anyone starting out on a diet (see Chapter 4). However, even in those people who don't achieve much in the way of weight loss with a low carb diet, there can still be a useful improvement in glucose levels and/or a reduced requirement for medications to control them.

However, low carb diets are not without their problems in people with type 2 diabetes, the most important of which may be the increased intake of fat that can sometimes occur when trying to avoid carbs, which can have unwanted effects on your lipid levels (see Chapter 8).

Some people can find that elimination of carbohydrate-rich foods from their diet also removes many of their favourite meals. This can lead to them feeling overly restricted with their new diet. For the same reasons, a low carb diet may also not suit vegetarians. On the plus side this may be one reason why people on a low carb diet eat less. However, it can also lead to many people breaking their diet and falling back into old habits.

Although you are eating fewer carbs, this does not necessarily mean you are more likely to experience dangerously low glucose levels (known as hypoglycaemia — see Chapter 7) when sticking to a low carb diet. However, the improvements in glucose control and weight loss that are achieved through changes in your diet can mean that if you are taking glucose-lowering medications that can sometimes cause hypoglycaemia, such as sulphonylureas or insulin, these may need to be reduced or stopped to prevent hypos. It could be said that a spoon *less* of sugar really does helps the medicine go down.

Sweeteners and sugar substitutes

Another popular way to reduce the total amount of sugar in your diet is to choose foods and beverages that substitute any sugar with a **sweetener**. Sweeteners can provide the sweet taste of sugar but have less or no effect on your glucose levels or the amount of energy you are getting from your food. This is the principle of many 'diet' drinks and low-energy products now on the market. These 'diet' products can be quite effective for people who get a lot of their dietary carbs from sweet foods or drinks.

The most commonly used sugar substitutes are **artificial sweeteners**, such as saccharin, aspartame and Acesulfame K. These have a very intense sweet taste when compared to table sugar, so can be used in very small amounts while producing a similar sweetness. Artificial sweeteners have minimal or no effect on blood glucose levels. In addition, the energy (calories) contained in diet products containing sweeteners can also be much less than that in regular products made with added sugars. And less energy in your diet means less fat will accumulate in your body. Importantly, when used in recommended amounts, artificial sweeteners appear to have no adverse effects on human health.

However sweet, though, the taste of artificial sweeteners is not quite the same as sugar. Sugar also contributes to the thickness or 'syrupiness' of a product, particularly a drink, so products with artificial sweeteners can sometimes feel 'thinner' in the mouth when compared to the usual sugar-laden products. To solve these dual problems of taste and bulk, many diet products are now made up of complex mixtures of artificial sweeteners and bulking agents, and achieve a reasonable approximation of a natural sweet sensation. This is harder to do on your own, so simply replacing table sugar in your house with artificial sweeteners may not be as practical or as tasty as it sounds. Also some of these artificial sweeteners break down when heated, so they can't be used in baking.

Another group of so-called 'natural sweeteners' has more recently emerged as a low calorie alternative to sugar, including **sucralose** (also known as Splenda®) and **stevia**. Some formulations of these products are stable when heated and can therefore be used for cooking and baking.

Sucralose is just ordinary table sugar (sucrose) that has been chlorinated. This makes it over 500 times as sweet as sugar, so you need 500 times less to achieve the same sweetness. Only 15 per cent of it is absorbed into the body (compared with nearly 100 per cent of sucrose) so its footprint on your glucose control is also very small.

Extracts of *Stevia rebaudiana*, a South American herb plant, are also increasingly used as natural sweeteners. Stevia is over 300 times as sweet as sugar, again meaning you need to use very little to get a sweet fix, and it contains no sugar and no food energy (calories).

The glycaemic index

It used to be believed that eating too many sweet things was the main reason for glucose levels to rise in people with diabetes. Consequently, the management of diabetes was all about not eating sweet things. Certainly, sweet foods and drinks often contain large amounts of simple sugars that are rapidly digested and absorbed. But many other foods also have the potential to release their sugars very quickly and cause your glucose levels to rise if enough insulin is not also quickly made and released.

Another approach to lower the load of glucose on the pancreas is simply to target just the quality of carbohydrate in your food. This is because the carbs contained in some foods have greater and faster effects on your glucose control than others. This effect can be measured as a food's **glycaemic index** or **GI** for short.

The glycaemic index scores different foods on how quickly and how much their carbs raise glucose levels when compared with eating the same amount of glucose. For example, a meal with a GI of 50 will raise the glucose levels by half as much as eating the same amount of glucose.

By convention, low GI foods have a GI of less than 55 (which means 55 per cent of the effect on glucose levels of eating an equivalent amount of glucose). Low GI products deliver their carbohydrate load slowly, so the demands on the pancreas to produce insulin are not so steep. This is why these low GI foods are sometimes called **slow carbs**.

Foods that have a GI greater than 70 are called high GI. The carbohydrate contained in these foods is digested and absorbed quickly. This causes a rapid surge of glucose into the blood and the requirement for an equally rapid surge in insulin production in response, to prevent blood glucose levels from rising. Interestingly, table sugar (sucrose) has a GI of around 60. Many sweet foods containing lots of table sugar have a lower GI than ordinary white bread or standard breakfast cereals. This means that they have less effect on your glucose levels. From the low GI standpoint, avoiding table sugar and foods that contain it may therefore be less important for your glucose control than tackling the high GI starches or things rich in corn syrup (which is rapidly broken down to release glucose that has a GI of 100).

The sweet sugar present in fruit and vegetables is called **fructose**. It has an even lower effect on glucose levels than table sugar, with a GI of around 20. Again, this means that foods made sweet by fruit, and fruit itself, generally have a low GI so need not be avoided by people with type 2 diabetes for better glucose control. And, of course, this creates many more opportunities for fashioning a new healthy, flavoursome diet.

The GI was originally developed to help people with diabetes improve their blood glucose control. In people with type 2 diabetes, producing large amounts of insulin rapidly is exactly what their pancreas can't do very well. This is one of the reasons why glucose levels rise more rapidly in people with diabetes after eating high GI foods, and why finding a low GI alternative is a good idea for glucose control in people with type 2 diabetes.

Low GI diets

Many people with type 2 diabetes are now recommended to go on a **low GI diet**, which simply aims to substitute any high GI products in your diet with low GI alternatives so that the carbs you do eat are mostly slow carbs. Again, this can be achieved in one of two ways. You can follow a low GI meal, recipe or menu plan in which the authors have already made sure the foods you will be eating are low GI. There are many that are suitable for people with type 2 diabetes including the 'New Glucose Revolution' diet books and the South Beach Diet. Alternatively, you can make a low GI diet yourself by finding out the GI of the foods you currently eat and then finding alternatives that have a slower glucose profile. At least initially, this requires you to check tables, books, websites and phone apps. These can give you an estimate of the GI of most foods and help you to choose the lowest GI alternative. Some products also display their GI proudly on their label. An example of some of the carb swaps you can consider include:

Common high GI food	Lower GI alternative
Puffed and flaked breakfast cereals	Unrefined cereals (e.g. bran)

Common high GI food	Lower GI alternative
White bread, bagels, buns	Wholegrain breads, sourdough, fruit loaf
Potato (especially baked, boiled or mashed)	Legumes, sweet potatoes, yam, sweet corn
White rice	Basmati rice, pearled barley, quinoa, pasta
White bread sandwich	Sushi (the stickiness means low GI)
Plain biscuits or crackers	Fruit

The reason why one product is low GI and another is high GI is complex and hard to predict. Low GI foods are not simply those with high fibre (although many are). For example, puffed wheat is high in fibre but also high GI. Equally, high GI foods are not all starchy or sweet (although many are).

The GI of food is influenced not only by the type of carbohydrate it contains but also its content of fat, protein, fibre and water. For example, protein and fat in foods can lower its GI by slowing its passage through the stomach and subsequent digestion. This means that some potato chips that are also high in fat can have a lower GI than baked potatoes.

The GI can also vary significantly between foods that look and taste the same. For example, some potatoes have a low GI while others have a GI greater than 100 (i.e. worse than eating straight glucose). This is why tables, books, phone apps etc. are so essential for making the most of a low GI diet. With practice you will come to know which foods increase your glucose levels and which ones don't, and can then make your choices accordingly.

But while each of these can be a good guide, the GI of any food is not static. The preparation and processing of a food (cooking method and time, amount of heat or moisture used, etc.) can change its GI. For example, although pasta falls into the low GI category, the more it is cooked the higher its GI becomes. For this and other reasons it is best to eat pasta *al dente* and not out of a tin. Drinking alcohol with meals can also lower your meal's GI by slowing the emptying of your stomach. The GI for a piece of fruit can also change as the fruit ripens or with prolonged storage.

The other important feature of GI is that only foods containing carbohydrate are given a score and GI only ranks food on their effect on glucose levels. It doesn't rank them based on how healthy they are for other things, such as fat or calories. For example, sausages are low GI but are often high in fat. Overall, a low GI diet should probably be best considered as only one part of an overall strategy of dietary change. But it is a good place to start.

These reservations aside, a low GI diet is a practical and potentially useful tool for the management of type 2 diabetes. It is relatively easily to achieve, perhaps more so than any other dietary intervention for the management of diabetes. It is not particularly restrictive, as it does not require you to avoid any category of food, or change your menu. It doesn't require you to reduce the volume of what you are eating or count carbs or calories (but you can as well if you want to lose weight). It also means that you don't end up eating more fat, which may be a problem for people with type 2 diabetes on a strict low carb diet.

There is also now good data to show that adherence to a low GI diet is able to improve glucose control in people with type 2 diabetes. Indeed, results have suggested that, in people with type 2 diabetes, the effect on glucose levels of sticking to a low GI diet is approximately equivalent to adding medications that specifically target blood glucose levels after meals. Low GI diets may also have beneficial effects on lipids, blood pressure and weight control.

Importantly, while glucose levels may fall if you go on a low GI diet, the risk of hypoglycaemia is not increased. In fact, it may be reduced as the slower delivery of glucose from low GI foods acts to maintain glucose levels for longer after meals, when glucose levels are usually at their lowest. By contrast, the rapid rise in glucose induced by high GI foods not only leads to high swings in glucose levels but can also lead to rebound lows as increased insulin released in response causes a much steeper fall in glucose levels.

High fibre diets

Another way to target carbohydrates is to focus on the amount of **fibre** in your diet. Fibre is only found in plants and their products. There is no fibre in meat, even if it is chewy. Fibre is the indigestible part of plant material (also known as **roughage**). Chemically, fibre is mostly made up of long chains (polymers) of sugars joined together so that they won't come apart when you eat them. This is why eating fibre has little or no effect on your glucose levels.

There are two types of dietary fibre: soluble and insoluble. Some fibre is able to dissolve in water. This is called **soluble fibre**. This kind of fibre is found in almost all plant foods. The highest amounts are found in legumes, such as lentils, beans and peas. Other excellent sources of soluble fibre include wholegrains (such as wheat, rye, oats, barley and brown rice), nuts and popcorn.

Some fibre tends to absorb water but does not dissolve in it. This is called **insoluble fibre**. This kind of fibre is most abundant in wholegrains. The highest levels are found in the outer husk of the grain, which is called the **bran**. Significant but lower levels of insoluble fibre are also found in nuts and seeds and refined cereals. Insoluble fibre is also found in the skins of vegetables and fruits, such as strawberries, prunes, tomatoes, apples, potatoes and onions.

The presence of soluble fibre in food slows its digestion and the subsequent absorption of glucose. Think about eating an apple compared to drinking apple juice. Of course, the same amount of juice will cause a greater rise in your glucose levels than just eating the apple. This is because soluble fibre transforms what you have just eaten into a sticky gel that releases its nutrients only gradually, making it less of a challenge for your insulin-producing capacity.

By holding food in your intestine for longer, a meal rich in fibre can also make you feel satisfied for longer when compared to an identical product devoid of its fibre. This means you may be less likely to feel hungry or need to snack between meals. A high fibre diet can also reduce the levels of harmful cholesterol in your blood (see Chapter 9).

In addition, fibre is also good for the health of your bowels and helps to prevent constipation, which is a common problem for people with type 2 diabetes. Fibre will act to absorb water, which makes your stool softer and more bulky. This makes it much easier for your bowels to push. However, if you increase the amount of fibre in your diet too quickly, or don't drink enough, fibre can actually cause constipation. If you double your fibre intake, you should generally also double your water intake.

All fibre is resistant to human digestion. But some fibre is digested by the bacteria of your large intestine, which releases gas. If you add fibre into your diet too quickly it can make you feel bloated and flatulent. This appears to be its only major drawback. So when ramping up the amount of fibre in your diet or using fibre supplements it is important to start slowly to allow your bowels and their bacteria to adjust to the change. Increasing your fibre intake gradually over a month until you reach your target should be sufficient.

Increasing the amount of fibre in your diet

All people with type 2 diabetes should aim for around 30g of fibre each day in their diet. Most adults eat less than half this amount.

There are a number of simple ways in which you can increase your intake of fibre. Many processed foods, such as bread and breakfast cereals, list their fibre content on the 'nutritional information panel'. In general, an excellent source of fibre will contain at least 5g per serve. A good source of fibre will contain more than 2.5g per serve. A product that claims to have added fibre will have at least 2.5g more per serve than if it wasn't added.

If you also want to go low carb (i.e. five to ten serves of carbs a day), you must ensure that almost all your carbs are coming from good or excellent sources of fibre to reach the recommended daily target of 30g.

Another way to increase the intake of fibre in your diet is to substitute products that use refined grains with **wholegrain alternatives**. These products retain either intact grains, flaked or 'cracked' grain kernels, coarsely ground kernels or use flour that is made from wholegrains (known as wholemeal flour). Milling or the refining of grains removes the germ and the bran (which contain most of the fibre) leaving behind only the inner starchy (high GI) part of the grain. For example, the amount of fibre in standard white flour is ten times lower than that of wholemeal flour.

Some simple ways to increase the amount of fibre in your diet include:

» Eat a breakfast cereal that lists 'wholegrain' or bran as the main (first) ingredient instead of one that contains just wheat. You should be able to find one containing at least 5g of fibre per serve. Alternatively, add a few tablespoons of bran to your favourite cereal. Brans are more concentrated sources of fibre, meaning you need to eat less to get the same amount.

» Switch white bread for wholegrain or wholemeal bread. Many breads contain some or all of these components, but they may not be truly wholegrain or high in fibre unless a wholegrain is the main (first) ingredient. Many breads are made brown because of added sugar (molasses) or are made to look healthy with a few scattered seeds. However, some products are fortified with significant amounts of added fibre. Again, most commercial breads will now list their nutritional contents on the label. So to select one that is a good source of fibre, choose one that has at least 2.5g of fibre per serve.

» For the same reasons, substitute some or all of the white 'all purpose' flour you use for your own baking with wholegrain wheat flour. You might need more yeast and baking powder to get your baking to rise, because wholemeal flour is heavier than traditional white flour. Also throw in some bran when you bake anything, from meatloaf to muffins and biscuits/cookies.

» Replace some or all of the white rice in your diet with brown rice. To make brown rice, only the husk is removed from the rice grain. But to make white rice, the brown coloured fibre-rich layers (the bran and the germ) are removed, again leaving behind only the inner starchy (high GI) part of the grain. This allows white rice to cook faster and fluff up nicely, but it also means that white rice contains four times less fibre than brown rice. Alternatively, throw in some barley with your white rice for some added fibre and flavour.

» Different kinds of wholewheat pasta are also now available as a substitute for standard white pasta. These can take a little getting used to because of their colour, nutty taste, texture and longer cooking time, which is about twice that of regular pasta. Some products are more palatable than others. But if you are making a good sauce, especially one that contains legumes, it is hard to tell the difference.

Just by replacing refined products with wholegrain equivalents, without changing anything else in your diet, you can more than double your intake of total and soluble fibre.

Other simple tricks to increase your fibre intake include:

» When making fruit juice, don't get rid of the skin and pulp. These are the good parts. Choose the whole fruit every time where possible.

» Don't peel off the skin from fruit, such as apples and pears, and vegetables such as carrots, potatoes, sweet potato and the pods of peas, as peeling them decreases their fibre content.

» For snacks, instead of processed carbs eat fruits with edible (whole) seeds, such as berries and kiwi fruit or fibre-rich fruits such as apples, pears, bananas, citrus and stone fruit. Vegetables with good soluble fibre content include

cauliflower, zucchini (courgettes), broccoli, carrots,
Jerusalem artichokes and celery.

» Substitute animal protein in your diet with legumes.
For example, use beans, chickpeas, lentils and soybeans
instead of some or all of your steak mince in your spaghetti
bolognese. Use legumes in your curry instead of some or all
of the meat. Again, these highly flavoured dishes mean that
the taste of the meal is not substantially changed, while its
fibre content is increased and fat content decreased.
A cup of red kidney beans will provide almost half your daily
fibre requirements. If you don't like beans you can also try
substituting other fibre-rich vegetables such as broccoli,
artichoke or Brussels sprouts.

For some people with diabetes, changing to a diet with large
amounts of wholegrain, bran and legumes is a major shift.
Another simple way to get fibre into your day without changing
what you eat too much can be to take fibre supplements.
These are available in many different forms, such as tablets,
capsules and powders (which can be mixed up as a drink). These
supplements don't provide the extra nutrients contained in
wholegrain products that may be beneficial to your health, but
they give you the fibre that may be lacking in your diet. It is also
important to remember that fibre supplements must be started
slowly and only gradually increased to your target intake over a
month. This will give your bowels a chance to adjust, in order to
reduce problems with bloating, flatulence and constipation.

4.

Waist management

UNDERSTAND

» The most important goal of changing your diet is to reduce the amount of fat in your body.

» Most weight loss diets focus on only one key component in your diet (calories, fat, carbs or GI), which makes them simple to follow and easy to stick to.

» There is no such thing as the best diet for weight loss. On average, most diets achieve about the same amount of weight loss of around 2 to 4kg (4½–9lb).

» It is likely that the mere process of embracing any dietary restrictions, thinking about and coordinating the foods you eat, makes you tend to eat less (energy) and eat better.

» Successful waist management is not all about changing *what* you eat; it also involves changing *how* you eat.

MANAGE

» Adopt a diet. It probably doesn't matter which one, so long as you enjoy it and are able to stick with it for the long term.

» Find out what you are eating. Explore the nutritional information guides on the foods that you currently eat, or download a program for your phone to help you do this on the fly.

» Start simply with realistic goals and small changes, and slowly work your way up to life-changing things.

» Get help from your doctor, dietician or other health professionals to find a diet that is best for you. Get help from your family. It's always hard to do just on your own.

The biggest health challenge of type 2 diabetes is not glucose control, but its direct antecedent, the accumulation of fat outside of where it is normally safely stored. This is usually associated with an expanded waistline.

Possibly the most important goal of changing your diet is to reduce the amount of fat in your body.

Long-term waist management is not only possible in people with type 2 diabetes but is also associated with a reduced risk of many of its complications. This can be achieved in many different ways, including regular exercise, medications and surgery. But the most common way to weight loss is through changing your diet.

Many of the things contained in your diet release energy as they are broken down by your metabolism. The amount of 'food energy' that is released can be measured and quantified as **kilojoules** or **calories**. (Note that 1 calorie is equal to approximately 4.12 kilojoules.) The different chemical components that make up your food release different amounts of energy when burnt by the body. For example, fats release twice as much energy when metabolised compared to protein or carbohydrate. In other words, fat and the products that are rich in fat contain more calories or kilojoules (of food energy).

Energy is too precious a thing for the body to waste. The equation is simple: if you eat it and you don't burn it immediately in your metabolism or physical activities, then you store it, mostly as fat. It does not seem to matter if you eat too many sweets or too many steaks, and you don't need repeated rounds of super-sized overconsumption. Usually there is only a small mismatch between the energy (calories) you get from your diet and energy used up by your metabolism and physical activity. This is known as a **positive energy balance**. Every time you run your energy balance into the positive, you get fatter.

Most adults will eat and drink well over 10,000kJ (2390 calories) of energy every day. However, their daily energy requirements will probably be more like 8000 to 9000kJ (1910–2150 calories). This is why so many people are getting slowly fatter as they get older and so many are getting diabetes.

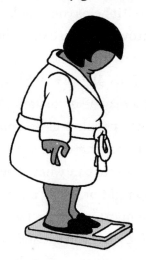

The object of changing your diet is not just to lose weight but to reduce the amount of fat in your body, especially around your waist.

Weight loss diets

The only way to get rid of the fat is to run a **negative energy balance**. This is partly achieved by reducing the amount of energy (calories) you get from food and drink each day while at the same time burning more energy by being physically active. It is a very simple equation, but sadly is not as simple to implement or maintain in a modern lifestyle.

Reducing the amount of energy (calories) you get from what you eat and drink can be successfully approached in any number of very different ways. There is no 'one size fits all' strategy. The most common way to try to reduce your energy intake is to go on a diet. This means regulating some or all of your entire food intake according to a plan. There are millions of diets out there. Each requires some adherence to a formula, recipe book or strategy for its success.

The media is full of inflated claims that one diet may be better than another, producing better weight loss because of a particular (magical) mix of nutrients. Whether the composition of a diet significantly affects how well it helps you to reduce the fat in your body remains highly controversial. Each has advantages and disadvantages. On average they will all achieve about the same amount of weight loss — 2 to 4kg (4½–9lb). However, on an individual basis their effects may be quite variable. Some diets that work really well for some people will be unpalatable or impossible for others. The fact that there are so very many diets out there that are so very different in what they let you eat should tell you that there is no right or wrong answer. What you are eating is probably not as important as the fact that you are sticking to some sort of plan for what you eat and are eating fewer calories. It is likely that the mere process of embracing any dietary restrictions, thinking about and coordinating the foods you eat, makes you tend to eat less (energy) and eat better. No matter how well it might work, if you can't stick with it, it's never going to give you what you want.

Overall, the best outcomes are probably seen when different approaches are used in combination. For example, it is often recommended that what best fits the bill to reduce weight is a combination of a low glycaemic index, low fat diet with increased soluble fibre and protein intake together with behavioural interventions, support measures and adjustment of diabetes medications. This may sound extraordinarily complicated but it is essentially a description of a basic, healthy diet.

Although most weight loss diets share a number of common elements, they can be divided into essentially four main categories:

» low calorie (or low energy) diets
» low fat diets
» low carbohydrate diets
» low GI diets.

Each of these diets chiefly focuses on changing only one particular component of your diet, without (directly) worrying about any others. This has the advantage of simplicity. As you've only got one thing to look out for, it also makes it easier to stick to.

It is beyond the scope of this book to describe any of these different approaches in the detail required to make them really work for you. This information can be easily found elsewhere, in books and magazines and on the internet. However, their broad characteristics can be summarised as follows.

Low calorie diets

Low calorie diets aim to directly limit your energy (calorie) intake. As far as low calorie diets are concerned, a calorie is a calorie no matter where it comes from. You make your choices on calories alone. It doesn't really matter what you are eating so long as it adds up to fewer calories in the end.

A low calorie diet can be achieved in essentially two different ways. The first method is to estimate how much energy (calories) is contained in everything you eat, and make a plan to restrict your diet based on a set number of calories at each meal or over a day. This is known as **calorie counting** and is widely practised by people wanting to lose weight and keep it off.

The first step in calorie counting is usually to work out how much energy you really need to be getting from your diet (known as the **daily energy requirement**). This can be calculated using the Harris Benedict principle, which takes into account your age, gender, size and level of activity:

Women: 655.1 + (9.56 × weight in kg) + (1.85 × height in cm) – (4.68 × age in years) × activity factor × 4.12 (if you want the result in kilojoules)

Men: 664.7 + (13.75 × weight in kg) + (5 × height in cm) – (6.76 × age in years) × activity factor × 4.12 (if you want the result in kilojoules)

Note: To work out your daily energy requirement in calories, leave out the 4.12 at the end of the calculation.

The activity factor in each equation (which adjusts for how active you are) is:

» for those who do little or no exercise each day, multiply by 1.2
» for those who do light exercise one to three days a week, multiply by 1.375
» for those who do moderate exercise three to five days a week, multiply by 1.55
» for those who do hard exercise six to seven days a week, multiply by 1.725
» for those who do daily exercise, a physical job or hard training, multiply by 1.9.

Let's say you are a 50-year-old woman who is 156cm tall and weighs 80kg. You're doing a little light exercise one to three days a week. Using this equation you can calculate that you need to eat about 8500kJ (2030 calories) of energy in your diet each day if you don't want to add any more fat to your body. But to get rid of fat you need to subtract energy from your diet and run in negative balance. You could step up your exercise level (which would mean that eating the same 8500kJ would now be 1000kJ less than your requirements, so you'd soon start losing weight). But if you just wanted to lose weight through your diet, a good place to start is with an energy deficit of about 500kJ (120 calories) each day. So in your calorie counting diet you'd plan to only eat 8000kJ (1910 calories) a day. This will generally achieve a weight loss rate of approximately 0.5kg (1lb) per week. Using this formula you can also appreciate how combining diet and increased physical activity is the easiest way to a negative energy balance and a slimmer waistline. But more on exercise in the next chapter.

After you have determined your target calorie intake, the next step in calorie counting is to work out how many calories are contained in the food you are eating. Some information can be obtained by reading the 'nutritional information panel' that is present on the labels of most processed foods. Look first at the **serving size** section. All the information below it will be about what you will get when you eat this amount of the product. If you eat more than this, which is usually the case with most of these products, all the nutrients you will also be getting will increase proportionally, including the calories. There are also many recipe books, websites and phone apps that are now available to provide useful information about how many calories are contained in most kinds of food and drinks, which can help in planning your meals.

For example, the energy in a packet of nacho chips is around 2000kJ (478 calories) per 100g (almost the same as butter) while most fruit and vegetables contain fewer than 400kJ (96 calories) per 100g. So if you are sticking to your plan of 8000kJ (1910 calories) a day, you can still have your energy-rich nachos, but that's a quarter of all the energy you can have that day. And this leaves less room for other things. But if you eat an apple instead, then you have more room for something else later. Unlike the other diets detailed below, this kind of diet can be quite flexible with what you eat. In fact it's largely your choice (e.g. whether you eat nachos or apples) so long as you stay within the limits imposed by the calorie count. The other advantage is that you quickly learn how to substitute foods that eat into your calorie count with those that eat into your waistline.

Another approach to limiting the energy contained in your diet is to follow a diet, meal or menu plan that swaps your intake of high calorie foods for products that carry less energy but have about the same volume and the same or more nutrients. The object is to make every mouthful contain less energy than it did before, while at the same time you get to eat the same satisfying portions. Two of the most commonly used low calorie diets are the DASH Diet and Weight Watchers.

Often the first thing a dietician will do to help you lose weight is to take a close look at what you are currently eating and find out which parts of your daily menu are providing you with excess energy. Rather than causing a major shift in your diet, often only a few targeted strikes can be all it takes to successfully reduce the energy content of your diet and the fat around your middle.

For example, soft drinks (sodas) and 'juices' represent major sources of excess energy. Over one-fifth of the sugar in a typical diet comes from these unnecessary drinks. The corn syrup sugars used in most soft drinks are the same as those in concentrated apple juice used in the bulk of fruit drinks. On average the energy in a can of Coke is around 500kJ (120 calories). So substituting all soft drinks in your diet for (low calorie) water can make a big difference to your waist. Many waist-conscious drinkers have also embraced diet versions which substitute sugar with other sweet chemicals and so contain less or none of the energy of their fully sugared parents. These sugar substitutes are discussed in detail in Chapter 3.

Another important cause for the excessive amounts of calories in our diet is so-called **energy-dense foods**. These contain a large amount of energy (calories) for their weight and are essentially concentrated energy. Some of the most energy-dense foods are high in fat. As noted above, fat contains twice the energy (calories) per gram when compared to protein or carbohydrate. Fat also doesn't dissolve in water so fatty foods tend to be drier, meaning that calories are tightly packed. One teaspoon of butter contains almost the same amount of energy as two cups of raw broccoli. Low calorie substitutes can usually be identified as foods that are both low in fat but high in water or fibre to provide weight and volume to food, but without additional calories.

However, it's not just fat that contributes to calories. Other components in your diet may be energy dense too, including those with a high sugar content (e.g. cakes, confectionery, dried fruit and some highly processed breakfast cereals). Again, the 'nutritional information panel' will give you some idea.

Even within food groups the energy density can vary quite a lot. For example, there are 420kJ (100 calories) in a quarter of a cup of raisins. The same amount of energy is contained in two cups of grapes.

A low calorie diet will substitute:

» lean cuts for fatty chops
» reduced fat dairy for whole milk
» skinless chicken for fried chicken
» apples for apple juice
» whole fruit for dried fruit

» lentils for mince

» salads and soups for muffins

» fruit for chips or crisps.

You might think that eating low energy foods would just make you hungrier and therefore want to eat more. But this is not true. On average, if you reduce the energy-dense foods you eat by a quarter, you will reduce your energy intake by a similar amount. In fact, it has been argued that energy-dense foods make you overeat because they are less filling and this means you eat more in the long term. So reducing the energy density of every mouthful usually means that you eat less (fewer calories) and lose waist.

Low fat diets

Some of the extra energy in your diet comes from the fat you eat. Fat contributes twice the energy per gram when compared with other nutrients. Fat also doesn't make you feel as full as other nutrients do, so you tend to eat more. Even if you are not counting calories, by assiduously avoiding fat, whatever you eat will usually contain less energy. For example, just choosing a leaner cut of meat can reduce the energy you get from your steak even if the amount you eat or the menu does not change.

So another popular way to lose weight is to focus solely on limiting the amount of fat in your diet, without worrying too much about anything else. These so-called 'low fat diets' are very popular for weight loss and are simple to follow because you only care about fat. Among the most famous are the Pritikin and Ornish diets, which can offer an effective means of weight loss for some, but not all, people.

Again, you can do this quite easily yourself by seeing how much fat is contained in the food you eat (based on the nutritional information panel) and choosing products with the lowest fat levels. Then you can simply substitute those things that contain animal fat (meat, milk, eggs, etc.) with low fat or vegetable alternatives. This is precisely what people on a low calorie diet are also doing, although for a different reason.

The other advantage of reducing the amount of fat in your diet is that you can also improve your lipid levels (see Chapter 9) along with your waistline. Many low fat diets also tend to have a high fibre content, which also helps with glucose control.

The major problem with low fat diets is that fat is not the only source of calories. Reducing the proportion of fat in your diet will not lead to weight loss unless the total amount of energy you are getting from your diet is also reduced (and exceeded by energy expenditure). Any extra energy from carbohydrates (sugar) or protein in your diet is still going to be converted and stored as fat. So overeating will still make you fatter, even if you are following a low fat diet. In fact, most people are eating much less fat than they did 20 years ago and yet the average size of their waistlines has not improved and, if anything, has got bigger.

It has also been argued that low fat diets may not be successful because when you get rid of fat in many of these low fat diet plans you often replace it with high GI carbohydrates, which potentially makes both glucose and weight control more difficult.

Low carbohydrate diets

As discussed in Chapter 3, diets low in carbohydrates are popular for the management of type 2 diabetes because of their beneficial effects on glucose control. However, low carb diets can also help in waist management.

The sole focus of low carb diets is to reduce your carbohydrate intake. You can do this yourself by estimating how many carbs are contained in different products and planning your meal and how much of it you will eat to match your chosen limit. This practice is known as **carbohydrate counting** or **counting carbs** and is widely used by people wanting to lose weight and keep it off.

Alternatively, you can begin a low carb diet, in which any foods that are high in carbohydrates are strictly limited or substituted with foods containing more proteins and/or more fats (e.g. meat, poultry, fish, shellfish, eggs, cheese, nuts and seeds). Some low carb diets just replace common carb-rich products with other foods that are essentially low in carbohydrates (e.g. non-starchy salad vegetables for potatoes or rice).

Perhaps the most well-known example of a low carb diet is the Atkins Diet. However, there are a range of other diets that share roughly the same principles with respect to carbs but vary in their relative amounts of other nutrients (e.g. how much fat or protein you eat). For example, the Atkins Diet does not restrict the fat you can eat, while the CSIRO Total Wellbeing Diet and the Zone Diet reduce both fat and carbohydrate in your diet, so the relative proportion of energy from protein goes up (which is why they are also sometimes called **high protein diets**). This can have the added effect of suppressing hunger and promoting your sense of fullness earlier in the meal.

Low carb diets tend to work faster than other weight loss plans. This is because the sugars stored in your body (as glycogen) are rapidly used up to make up for the carbs you are not getting from your diet. The chemical release of glycogen from its stores uses up water. So although your weight quickly falls within a week, which is a great positive reinforcement, you mostly lose water. It may be that excess fat is not removed which, after all, is the primary goal of your diet. The other problem comes if you fall off the wagon and return to your normal diet. As you are now eating more carbs, your body is able to put away more glucose stores, which releases water. This means that your weight can very quickly rebound, even if you are not actually getting fatter. Therefore your weight could yoyo on a low carb diet more than with other strategies, as faithfulness to your diet rises and wanes.

Low GI diets

Another practical approach to waist control is to go on a **low GI diet**, which only considers how quickly a food will cause a rise in blood glucose levels (known as the glycaemic index or GI). It does not concern itself with the amount of carbs or calories you are eating, but rather the kind of carbs you are taking in. A low GI diet aims to substitute any high GI products in your diet with low GI alternatives that deliver their carbohydrate at a slower pace. An example of some possible substitutions are provided in Chapter 3.

Because it is hard to predict why one product is low GI and another is high, a low GI diet relies (at least initially) on tables, recipe books, websites and apps that provide an estimate of the GI of most foods and help you to choose the lowest GI alternative. Some products also display their GI proudly on their label.

The real value of low GI diets in glucose control for people with type 2 diabetes is discussed in detail in Chapter 3. However, it is also clear that simply targeting the kind of carbohydrates you eat without doing anything else is enough to help you lose weight and keep it off. Eating predominantly low GI foods is the basis of many effective weight loss programs including the South Beach Diet and New Glucose Revolution Diet.

It is thought that high GI foods don't make you feel as full as other foods, or if they do it wears off more quickly and you're left feeling hungry again sooner. By contrast, the slow delivery of sugars from low GI foods keeps you satisfied for longer (known as **satiety**), which means you are less likely to want to eat again soon. This also means you tend to eat less between meals, which helps reduce your energy (calorie) intake.

Meal replacements

As an alternative to organising your own diet it is now possible to get someone else to do it for you by providing meal replacements and/or pre-packaged meals. For example, one or two of your meals each day can be effectively replaced with a low energy drink or bar that has an energy content of no more than 1000kJ and consists mostly of protein with a small amount of fat and carbohydrate. Some meal replacement programs provide frozen meals that you just defrost on the right day at the right time and eat. If you eat their food instead of relying on your own random habits, you are almost guaranteed to be eating less.

Meal replacement strategies have proved more successful for weight loss than trying to limit your calories across all your meals. This has made meal replacements some of the most popular and successful (in the short term) of all commercial weight loss plans. All you need to do is not fall off the wagon.

Their key limitation is the lack of flexibility with many programs, limited food choice and predictability of diet plans. Many do not include an education component, so that when the program is completed you haven't learnt self-reliance. Waist management in type 2 diabetes is a lifelong task not a temporary fad. Ideally, diets and meal replacements should be considered a great kick-start to your weight-loss program, which sees you ultimately take control of what you eat.

Changing eating behaviours

Successful waist management is not just about changing what you eat; it also involves changing *how* you eat. Changing eating behaviours and assuming control over what you are eating (even if it is only one component of your diet) appears to be pivotal for the long-term struggle to keep excess fat out of your body. The desire and momentum to keep new habits in place come from the individual.

The single most important factor in determining the success of any weight loss diet is whether you can stick with it for the long term.

To make healthy behaviours stick, it is also important to change your focus from the negative 'I can't eat that' to the positive 'I can have these'. Eating is one of life's great pleasures. When you shop, when you cook, when you eat, it is possible to get satisfaction from your diet without excess calories.

For a diet to be successful it cannot be considered a punishment that you have to endure in order to get healthy. That will never work. So the only real solution is if at first you don't succeed, try, try again until you find something that both works and that you enjoy — then run with it.

Even if you never change what you eat, or never follow a diet as such, it is possible to reduce the amount you eat by changing the way you eat. One simple trick is to leave one in every four behind. For example, for every four spoons of cereal you would have, eat three and leave one behind. For every four potatoes you'd eat, eat three and leave one behind. On its own, this technique is challenging, as smaller portions can leave you hungry and dissatisfied. So the combination of more filling (less energy dense) foods and reduced portion sizes is better than either on its own.

Another simple trick is to use smaller plates and bowls. When presented with larger portions most people generally just eat it all up, as hunger and fullness signals are overridden by the cue to clean the plate. To stop yourself overfilling, and make it look as if you are eating more than you really are, just use a smaller plate.

One of the important reasons we often eat is simply because food is there. That is how the human brain works. So plan your environment to support waist management. But rather than having a house devoid of food, make it easier to access fruit, vegetables and salads in your home and harder to get to the carbs, sweets, biscuits/cookies and chips.

The more often you eat, the greater the chance you will take in more energy (calories). It is obvious that every calorie outside of meal times is probably a calorie in excess. However, skipping meals is not a good solution. In fact, there is good data showing that regular eating patterns help waist control. For example, breakfast gets you going and makes you feel nourished and satisfied, and less likely to overeat for the rest of the day. Missing breakfast means you have less energy and makes you hungrier for snacks or larger portions at other meals, so you are always chasing your tail when it comes to glucose control.

Snacks

It is sometimes said that snacking between meals can prevent overeating due to excessive hunger. Certainly, some diet programs allow for snacks to help manage hunger and reduce bingeing. But it is usually not necessary to snack and any means to reduce the amount you are eating is worthwhile if you have type 2 diabetes. If you just have to snack, the trick is to make sure that these snacks don't add much to your energy balance. The best example is to reach for fresh fruit or vegetables (such as carrots or broccoli) when you snack instead of a sandwich, muffin or cake.

A more practical solution is to get a handle on when you are usually feeling the urge to snack. Is it mid morning, mid afternoon or in the evening? Once you know, you can try adding in more slow carbs to the meal immediately beforehand, to try to cover this period much better and reduce your hunger cravings.

Comfort food

One way many people cope with stress in their lives is by eating. If you are depressed, anxious, strung out, angry or filled with other negative emotions, food can be a comfort, hence the term 'comfort food'. The more stress you have in your life, the more you might look to offset it by eating. And it works, but only for a moment. Eating food will reliably alter mood and emotion, typically making you less grumpy and more calm, possibly by modifying brain function and triggering the release of 'calming' hormones. What is important in stress-related eating is to deal with the stress at the same time you are trying to lose weight (see Chapter 16). This makes it more likely that both will get better.

Setting weight loss goals

One of the most important components of a weight loss program is setting clear and achievable goals. Unrealistic expectations concerning weight loss frequently result in failure. Having a relevant and achievable target in front of you hardens your resolve and focuses your attention (not just 'I want to be thinner'). As an initial target it is recommended that those who are overweight should aim to reduce their current weight by 5 to 10 per cent (e.g. if you are 100kg/220lb, aim to initially reduce your weight to between 90 and 95kg/198 and 209lb). This might seem very small, but even this amount may be associated with improved health if it can be sustained.

It is also useful to keep a food diary or journal, recording everything you are eating. You can use either a book or a phone app for this. It is not simply a good way to see how you are tracking; some studies have shown that people who keep a daily food diary lose more weight than those who don't. Again, it appears that the act of paying close attention to what you are eating, and recognising that your choices actually matter, seems to be a key part of achieving weight loss.

Finally, waist control is not easy at the best of times. It can be even harder on your own. There are many providers out there who can offer advice and support. The most successful programs involve a strong relationship and long-term interaction between provider and consumer, be that a dietician, trainers, counsellors, motivators, a weight loss group or even your friends and family. So get some help!

Other options for management of the extremely overweight

In many people with type 2 diabetes, getting rid of excess fat can be achieved through keeping to a diet and increased physical activity. However, in some people who are dangerously overweight, medications and surgery are now available to make it easier to lose weight and improve health and wellbeing.

Orlistat is a medicine that reduces the absorption of fat from the diet by one-third, by inhibiting the enzymes that break down fats in the intestine. It was derived from a natural inhibitor of digestion found in bacteria. By limiting the amount of fat digested, orlistat also reduces the energy obtained from fat in your diet. In some individuals this is enough to cause a modest reduction in weight. However, many people cannot tolerate orlistat because of its side effects, including flatulence and oily, loose stools.

Phentermine and diethylpropion are **appetite suppressants**, chemically related to amphetamines, that work by changing the balance of neurochemicals in the brain to help you feel full after meals. Again, their effects are modest at best and they may be associated with significant side effects, including behavioural changes, anxiety, increases in heart rate and blood pressure. There is also a potential for dependence so they can only used for short-term treatment.

A number of different complementary herbal weight loss supplements are sold in health shops and claim to promote weight loss. None of these therapies has been proven to be consistently effective and some are actually dangerous depending on what they contain and how they are used.

By contrast, weight loss surgery (know as **bariatric surgery**) is a very effective means to produce sustained weight loss in severely overweight individuals. In many people, the weight loss is so significant that they become free of diabetes. The most common bariatric surgery techniques are **gastric banding**, **gastric bypass** and **gastric sleeve** surgery. All these surgical techniques require adherence to diet and exercise regimens for the full benefits to be achieved and sustained.

Gastric banding (also known as a **lap-band**) places an adjustable band around the upper part of the stomach, creating a small pouch. This pouch is smaller than a whole stomach and means you eat much less at any one time before feeling full. In the long term this means you eat smaller portions and lose weight over time. The size of the pouch can be individually adjusted so that it prevents overeating, but not so small as to prevent adequate nutrition. Because no part of the stomach is removed, the signals for hunger sometimes remain. However, by feeling full more quickly and for a longer period of time, this can lead to significant weight loss over time in some individuals. Weight loss with lap-banding also requires adherence to dietary changes to be successful.

Gastric bypass surgery also creates a small upper pouch that reduces the amount you can eat at one time, but it also surgically connects the small intestine to the new pouch, bypassing the remainder of the old stomach which is then removed. This means less hunger and better weight loss. However, it requires more complicated invasive major surgery, but bypassing the upper intestine has more significant effects on blood glucose control, with at least three out of every four people with type 2 diabetes who undergo this procedure not needing to take glucose-lowering medication anymore.

An intermediate form of gastric surgery thins the stomach to form a tube (known as a gastric sleeve) rather than a restrictive pouch. The part of the stomach that regulates hunger is also removed. This kind of surgery is more effective at producing weight loss than lap-banding, but may be less effective than gastric bypass surgery in terms of its effects on diabetes.

5.
Get physical

UNDERSTAND

» One-third of adults undertake no vigorous activity at all, or only now and then in very small/short doses. Most of their waking hours are spent sitting.

» People who sit for long periods are at greater risk of weight gain and have worse blood glucose and blood pressure control, no matter how much physical exercise they subsequently do.

» The health benefits of regular physical activity are far greater than the total amount of energy burnt, and are seen regardless of whether or not you lose weight.

» The stresses and strains that tax the body during vigorous exercise cause it to adapt. These adaptations are what is known as 'getting fit' and include better blood glucose, lipid and blood pressure levels.

» The same health benefits of physical activity can be achieved whether performed as a structured daily session (exercise) or as unstructured activity spread over the course of a day.

MANAGE

» Take all the little opportunities to be more active every day. Accumulate moderate-intensity physical activity in everyday tasks.

» Undertake a careful screening assessment of your health and fitness before commencing any new exercise program.

» Plan exercise as part of your regular daily commitments, rather than as an optional 'add on' to do 'when you have time'.

» Set yourself modest but realistic goals and keep updating them as you get fitter.

» Combine aerobic training with anaerobic exercises such as resistance training for added benefits with respect to fat burning and glucose control.

» Get help. People generally have greater success with exercise when they have supervision and encouragement from someone else, be that an exercise physiologist, trainer or a local club.

Most people don't get enough physical activity. This is not because they don't go to the gym, jog or lift weights. It is not because they are lazy. In fact, most people are far too busy; too busy, that is, to undertake any sustained vigorous activity on any regular basis. Such people are known as sedentary. Most of their busy waking hours are spent sitting at a desk, in a car, around the meal table or recovering from their day on the couch. Think about what you did yesterday: there's a good chance you too spent at least eight to ten hours sitting down.

While it may seem innocuous enough, this sedentary lifestyle is a killer. For example, when compared to those who undertake regular physical activity, inactive people have, on average, twice the risk of heart attacks. The magnitude of this effect is similar to being a smoker.

Type 2 diabetes is strongly linked to inactivity. People who engage in little physical activity are more likely to get type 2 diabetes even without an expanding waistline. Yet recognising that one reason you're sitting in the pickle jar of diabetes is because of sitting on your backside far too often makes the potential solution all the more apparent and urgent. Diabetes means it's time to get physical.

Of all the things that can be done to manage your diabetes, getting more physical activity is one of the most important. *You can have the best diet and take all your medication as prescribed, but if you remain inactive many of their benefits can be lost*

By contrast, the impact of diabetes and its complications can be reduced by just increasing your level of regular physical activity, often only very slightly. Engaging in regular exercise can also enhance the success of other initiatives, such as those aiming to control your blood glucose levels, your waistline, your blood pressure or lipid levels. When it comes to diabetes, if you really want to survive you need to get fitter.

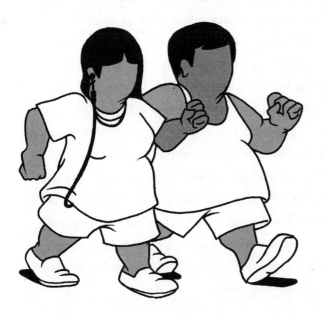

Of all the things that can be done to manage type 2 diabetes, physical activity is one of the most useful and most important.

Why do fit people survive?

There is good evidence that physical exercise has a number of direct and indirect effects on the human body that promote health and wellbeing.

Exercise burns energy

The most obvious reason for this is that exercise burns energy (calories) accrued from your diet that would otherwise be deposited as fat around your waistline. Consequently, alongside healthy nutrition, regular exercise is an important means to achieve and maintain weight control and to improve the body's composition. However, the health benefits of physical activity are far greater than the total amount of energy burnt, and are seen regardless of whether or not you lose weight when you exercise.

Exercise offsets insulin

When you are physically active, your muscles burn different kinds of fuel. The first fuel to be used is stored in the muscles themselves. Once exercise has burnt these stores, to keep going glucose is released into the bloodstream by the liver, and fat breakdown is increased so that it can also fuel the muscles. Your muscles then take up, burn and break down fats and glucose from the blood, which provides the energy for your muscles to contract and get their job done. After exercise is finished your muscles continue to take up large amounts of fat and glucose from the bloodstream to replenish their fuel stores in preparation for their next exertion. This uptake of glucose, both during and after exercise, can be very useful for people with type 2 diabetes, as it means less work for insulin and any medications. It also means less fat around your waistline.

Exercise triggers adaptations

The stresses and strains that tax the body during exercise cause it to adapt. These adaptations are what is known as 'getting fit' or 'the training effect'. Fitness includes adaptations in the heart, circulation, muscle, nerve and hormonal functions that vary according to the level and duration of physical activity. Precisely because it is taxing, exercise stimulates and adapts the body in ways that make you better able to cope with your next physical activity. However, these adaptations also have spin-off effects on many other aspects of your health, including those associated with diabetes and its complications. For example, muscles that are regularly used will adapt to become bigger and stronger, meaning they can do more next time with less effort and less fatigue at the end of it. At the same time, bigger muscles are also more efficient at taking up and burning glucose, which is a bonus for diabetes control.

The same sort of thing happens in your heart. Following regular exercise, the heart also becomes bigger and stronger, making it more able to provide the extra blood flow required to fuel your exertions. However, a stronger heart is a bonus for people with type 2 diabetes, who often experience reduced function of their heart. A strong heart also means a slower pulse and lower blood pressure.

Benefits from fitness are also seen in your feet. For example, type 2 diabetes can sometimes lead to reduced blood flow to your feet, which can have serious complications for your health (see Chapter 12). Regular exercise demands better blood flow to the legs to allow the muscles to work better. So the blood vessels supplying your legs progressively adapt to regular exercise to improve this blood flow. And if you have diabetes, this may be just what your feet need to stay healthy.

To trigger each of these adaptations, you have to undertake activities that tax each system. The heart must be pushed and the muscles must be tired. Not too hard, but enough to make these systems want to improve, to be better able to cope with future requirements; in essence, to get fitter.

Exercise improves risk factors

It is still possible to improve your health as a result of increasing your physical activity levels without necessarily being bigger, stronger or faster. For example, when people with type 2 diabetes perform regular exercise they can also reduce risk factors for complications such as high cholesterol, glucose and blood pressure levels without noticeably improving traditional markers of fitness, such as strength or endurance. Nonetheless, the greatest improvements are seen in those who can also achieve and sustain a level a physical fitness.

Exercise makes you feel good

Feeling well each day is an important part of diabetes management, and exercise is also good for the mind. Physical activity improves many aspects of psychological health, including self-esteem and emotional wellbeing. Exercise also lessens the impact of stress on your mood and your body, partly by modifying the synthesis or release of stress-response chemicals in the brain. It also works in preventing depression and in its treatment (see Chapter 16).

Exercise not only makes you feel better but also makes you think better. Exercise increases levels and the availability of chemicals that have protective benefits for several diseases of the brain. Exercise also directly enhances the capacity for learning and memory and slows their losses associated with age.

In addition, regular exercise improves the quality of your sleep, which is extremely beneficial for how you feel (see Chapter 17).

The problem with too much sitting

Finally, the reason why couch potatoes have such poor health outcomes is not simply because they are missing out on the health benefits of exercise. While it might feel comfortable, sitting down all day every day turns out to be directly damaging to your health. This is particularly the case where sitting is unbroken for long periods (on the computer, at the desk, in front of the television, etc).

People who sit for long periods are at greater risk of weight gain and have worse blood glucose and blood pressure control, no matter how much physical exercise they subsequently do. It is thought that because your muscles are inactive when sitting, more of the burden of metabolising the food you eat is placed on the pancreas (which in the setting of diabetes is having a hard time coping anyway!). So more of the energy (calories) in the diet of inactive couch potatoes ends up in the fat around their waistlines, instead of being burnt while moving your muscles. By contrast, staying on your feet at every opportunity, and breaking up long periods of sitting by getting up frequently, may be as important as engaging in a structured exercise such as going to the gym. For example, people who sit for fewer than 4 hours per day but don't exercise, appear to be at least as healthy as those who exercise at least 5 hours per week but spend most of their day sitting down.

Increasing your daily activity

There are many different ways to live a more active life. The same health benefits of physical activity can be achieved whether you are doing a structured daily session (exercise or training) or just making it up over the course of your day, as part of your life or your job.

The important part is simply being active on a regular basis, and to stop being a couch potato.

Many people can 'accumulate' the moderate-intensity physical activity they need in everyday tasks, such as:

» walking the kids to school
» walking or cycling to work
» taking the stairs instead of the lift
» getting off the bus one stop earlier and walking home
» parking a little further away and walking the difference
» speaking to colleagues in person rather than sending an email
» getting up and collecting your printing rather than waiting for someone to bring it to you
» breaking up your sitting time at least every half an hour; just standing up regularly uses your muscles and expends excess energy; the less you sit around the more healthy you can become.

Rather than being time-consuming or restrictive, taking every opportunity to put a little more physical activity into your day can be quite creative and invigorating. It requires little or no planning. The most exciting thing is that there are an endless number of options to try. The only thing that is limiting is taking the time to get up and get going.

However, the most familiar form of physical activity is exercise, which is any activity that is structured, planned and repetitive.

Doing exercise is probably the easiest way to ensure you engage in enough physical activities to build your health and resilience against diabetes and its complications.

Some form of exercise is generally required to become really fit. A good strategy is to plan exercise as a part of your regular daily commitments, rather than have it as an optional 'add on' to do 'when you have time'. Exercise sessions can be structured into a weekly work and recreation schedule to ensure they become a regular habit.

There are many different kinds of exercise, from walking and swimming, yoga and Pilates, to sports and more formal programs in a gym. Exercise broadly falls into two main categories: aerobic and anaerobic. Each has its own benefits and limitations, and the greatest benefits are probably gained when you do some of both over the course of your week.

Aerobic exercise

Aerobic exercise simply means doing some sort of physical activity that burns fuel in your muscles, using oxygen as the catalyst, to provide the energy required for movement. Aerobic exercise involves activities performed at moderate levels of intensity for extended periods of time.

Most continuous activities of more than 3 minutes are aerobic exercises, such as brisk walking, jogging, cycling, swimming, rowing, dancing, aerobics, as well as sports such as football, soccer, squash and tennis. They're all good. The best one for you depends on your interests and enjoyment, but mostly whether you can stick with it.

A number of studies have demonstrated the health benefits of just brisk walking on a regular basis. For example, a regular brisk walking program can improve your fitness, lower your blood pressure, improve your blood lipid profile and lower your blood glucose levels. This is often the easiest way to take up exercise. It is simple, cheap and right there at the end of your legs. For example, when compared to doing nothing at all, some health benefits can be observed with as little as 1 to 2 hours of walking at a moderate pace every week. This is a good place to start and may be all you can do or fit in. It might include walking for pleasure, walking the dog, walking to work or the shops or walking as a break from work. After a while it will get easier and you'll find yourself walking further, faster and more often. This soon adds up to better fitness and to better health outcomes.

Pedometers that count each step (by registering impacts as your feet hit the ground) can provide a simple method to assess your current activity, as well as a motivational tool to become more active. Sedentary people will generally accumulate fewer than 5000 steps a day. Although everyone should have their own target based on their age and level of fitness, a general goal should be to try to walk at least 10,000 steps every day (as publicised by Central Queensland University's 10,000 Steps program: http://www.10000steps.org.au).

It is recommended that all adults with type 2 diabetes should undertake some kind of regular, **moderate-intensity aerobic exercise** on 3 to 5 days of each week — not just on the weekend. Physical activity is best spread out across the week so that there is no longer than 2 or 3 days between each session. Ideally you should get some activity on most days. In total, you should aim to get at least 2 to 3 hours of aerobic exercise across every week, divided into sessions of about 30 to 45 minutes each.

Each session can be further divided into smaller blocks of 10 to 15 minutes each, with a rest period of 5 minutes between each segment or spread at intervals through the day to fit your exercise into your daily routine. As your fitness improves, the duration of each segment can gradually become longer or the rest period between each segment can become shorter. However, you have to ease into it. If you've been inactive for a while you can't go hard at it immediately. Some tips on getting started are listed later in this chapter.

Although the first target is 2 to 3 hours per week, better health outcomes are seen with longer and more frequent workouts; again, you have to build up to this. But while more is better, even a small increase in your level of activity provides some protection and benefit when compared to doing nothing at all.

The exercise you choose doesn't need to be very hard. But it needs to be enough to tax you and your muscles. This is called moderate-intensity exercise and is the goal of your aerobic exercise. But how intense this really is will be very different in different people. There are a number of different ways to judge this. For example, you can use a simple scale:

» level 0 is sitting down
» level 10 is the highest level of effort possible
» to exercise at moderate intensity you need to aim for 5 or 6.

If your exercise program is under the care of professional trainers, they will often determine the best program for you based on formal measures of your fitness. This can also be used to track your progress and provide quantitative motivational goals.

One of the most common tests of fitness is the VO2 max (also known as aerobic capacity, endurance exercise potential). This test is done by putting you through a graded exercise on a treadmill, bike or rowing machine (often referred to as an ergometer). The test starts easy and gets harder and harder until you reach your limits. While you are working away, the volume and composition of air breathed is directly measured, and how much oxygen you have used is calculated. Moderate-intensity activity should see you exercising at about 60 per cent of your VO2 max.

Another common way to judge the required intensity of an activity is to check your heart rate. When you start any physical activity, your heart rate will increase; the greater the intensity of the activity, the greater the increase in your heart rate. A rough guide to establishing an appropriate training intensity is to work at around 60 to 70 per cent of your age-adjusted maximal heart rate.

Your maximal heart rate can be estimated using the following formula:

Maximum heart rate = 220 minus your age (in years).

So if you are 60 years old, your maximal heart rate should be around 160 beats per minute. Then when you are exercising at moderate intensity, your heart should be racing at around 60 to 70 per cent of this figure, or between 100 and 112 beats per minute. This is also known as getting into 'the zone'. Many people find this the most convenient way to get a good aerobic workout.

It is important to note that these formulae apply only to healthy people and cannot be applied to those with heart disease and on certain medications that slow the heart. When prescribing appropriate exercise intensity, a number of other factors must also be taken into consideration, including age, health status, and current fitness and activity levels. Consequently, all those with diabetes should seek advice from their GP, an accredited exercise physiologist or a suitably qualified allied health professional, to set a target that is just right for them (see 'Starting an exercise program' on p. 83).

Although aerobic exercise is associated with improved health and wellbeing in people with type 2 diabetes, it does have some limitations when performed on its own. While aerobic training increases the capacity of the heart and lungs it may not have much effect on muscle strength or bone mass, both of which buffer the impacts of diabetes. Aerobic exercise also may not use up as much extra fat and glucose when compared to the same amount of strength training, although it can be undertaken for longer periods and more frequently to make up any difference. On the whole, aerobic exercise is best used as one component of a balanced exercise program that also involves some anaerobic exercises.

Anaerobic exercise

The phrase 'anaerobic exercise' describes undertaking short bursts of intense exertion at nearly 100 per cent effort, like sprinting or weight lifting. Because the energy required for this kind of activity is at or above the maximal ability to supply oxygen to the muscles, anaerobic exercise must rely on fuel stores already present within the muscles themselves. These stores are limited and maximal exertion cannot be sustained for more than 2 to 3 minutes before exhaustion sets in. But by specifically burning these muscle stores, anaerobic exercises set in motion adaptations that build strength, endurance and size of muscles. However, its success does not require you to become bulky or muscle-bound.

By exhausting your muscles' fuel stores, they respond by filling up again on glucose and fat which is drawn out of the bloodstream. And this means less work for insulin and often less medication.

The workload on the body during this kind of exercise is much higher when compared with that during aerobic exercise, like jogging or swimming. This means anaerobic exercise will be able to burn more energy and can have a greater impact on your metabolism and fat stores. However, it also means that special precautions must be taken by those with diabetes when undertaking this kind of exercise program (see below).

Strength training

Strength or **resistance training** is the best known form of anaerobic exercise. This is where your muscles move against an opposing force that resists their movement (known as resistance). The force resisting you may be the force of gravity (e.g. weights, push-ups and squats), elastic resistance (e.g. rubber tubing) or hydraulic resistance as used in many exercise machines.

For your resistance training to be effective you must do enough in a session to fatigue your muscles.

Generally, muscles are repeatedly worked at 65 to 75 per cent of their maximal capacity (known as **one repetition maximum or 1RM**) until the point of fatigue. This usually means 8 to 12 repetitions of a specific activity, which is called a **set**. To maximise the benefits, the last few repetitions of each set are supposed to be hard. If you can do more than 12 repetitions of the exercise then you are not using enough resistance.

When starting out, one set of each exercise is all that is required. This is gradually built up to three sets of each exercise, with a recovery period of 1 to 2 minutes between each set, to provide the best stimulus to increase muscle strength.

The beauty of such programs is that they are self-adjusting. Even if you have little strength, activities can be planned to be in keeping with your 1RM. As the body strengthens and adapts it will become easier to lift the same weight, so the applied resistance must be progressively increased to ensure you are continually strengthening your muscles and maximising the benefits of the exercise. This is usually done by gradually increasing the training intensity, duration, frequency, time or a combination of some of these parameters. For example, if you do not want to increase a weight, slowing the exercise down will increase the amount of work you are doing.

There are a number of different programs available. A strength program would generally consist of 8 to 10 different exercises that are specifically chosen to increase the strength of a range of muscle groups, but in particular the large muscles of the legs, buttocks, trunk and upper back.

Strength training is best conducted at least 2 or 3 times each week, on alternate days so the muscles have a chance to regenerate and become stronger as a result of repeated sessions. If you want to do your strength training every day, it is advisable to split the program into two segments (e.g. upper body on Monday, Wednesday and Friday and lower body on the Tuesday, Thursday and Saturday) so each muscle group has two days to recover between each session.

When undertaking a strength program it is important that each exercise is performed with the correct technique and that this is maintained throughout the set. This is known as **form**. This ensures that any activity achieves its desired outcomes and is performed safely. Loss of form, especially at the end of a set when muscles are tiring, not only reduces the effectiveness of an exercise but may also be dangerous.

Interval training

While aerobic fitness relies on continuous activity, additional fitness gains can also be achieved in already active people by alternating short bursts of vigorous exertion with intervals of lower activity. This is known as **interval training**. Interval training is not overly difficult and can be built up gradually according to your individual requirements. It may, for example, involve incorporating short periods of jogging as part of a basic walking program and progress to including multiple sprints of 100 to 200 metres with alternate periods of walking or jogging. Swimmers may include a couple of faster laps followed by slower laps. The high-intensity phase should be long enough and strenuous enough that you are out of breath by the end. Recovery periods (the slower, less intense periods of exercise) should be only long enough to result in a partial recovery before the next faster interval is begun. You should start with 10 to 15 minutes of warming up, followed initially by burst–recovery repeats totalling some 15 to 20 minutes, then end with a 10- to 15-minute period of cooling down. This is performed as part of training 2 or 3 times a week.

Interval training is more effective in burning fat than sustained moderate-intensity activity for the same or longer period. However, interval training is certainly more strenuous than continuous aerobic training, and generally requires increased levels of motivation. It should only be attempted by already active people and, in the context of diabetes, under the supervision of a doctor or appropriately trained exercise instructor.

Flexibility training

Although flexibility training (stretching exercises, yoga) has no direct effect on glucose control, it does help to improve and maintain the range of motion of your joints. This allows you to participate more easily, and with less pain, in other activities that can improve your health. As a result most programs also incorporate an element of flexibility training, in addition to aerobic and anaerobic components.

Starting an exercise program

Whenever you plan to start a new exercise program, it is important to take it slowly and stick within your limits. If you are getting started after a period of inactivity, exercising on alternate days is a good place to begin, with a day of recovery between each exercise day. The recovery days may also be used to incorporate another exercise type, such as strength or flexibility training.

The pre-assessment

While regular physical activity has an enormous number of benefits for those with diabetes, it also has risks. This is not a reason to remain a couch potato, but the demands of exercise may be different in different people. To ensure that any risks are minimised and to allow for appropriate exercise prescription, it is recommended that all those with type 2 diabetes undertake a careful screening assessment of their health and fitness before commencing any new exercise program. This may be conducted by a doctor, diabetes educator or exercise specialist. However, everyone in your diabetes care team should be updated on your plans, as exercise potentially impacts all aspects of diabetes care, from your feet to your mind and everything in between.

People with well-controlled diabetes or stable heart conditions do not need formal medical clearance before beginning a low to moderate physical activity program. However, it is essential for all those with complications, those with difficult diabetes management, and in those who are unsure as to their risks. The kind of things a pre-assessment will look out for include risks for 'hypos', heart disease, high or low blood pressure, and foot damage.

Risks for hypos

During and after exercise, blood glucose levels can fall as muscles draw in glucose from the bloodstream. This is why exercise is so effective in controlling glucose levels in diabetes.

The majority of people with type 2 diabetes have glucose levels that are high enough to buffer the effects of exercise. However, some of the medicines that lower glucose levels in people with type 2 diabetes have the potential to cause **hypoglycaemia** when combined with exercise. The solution is not to avoid exercise, but to plan it better with the help of your diabetes care team. For the minority who do experience these 'hypos' with exercise, they can be mostly prevented by better coordinating their physical activity with their medication. For example, not exercising straight after taking your medication can be useful. Some people also find it useful to carry some carbohydrate-rich snacks which they can eat in case they get caught up in physical activity that is more vigorous or more prolonged than originally planned. Another strategy is to eat your snack if glucose levels are already less than 5.6mmol/L (100.8mg/dL) before starting your activity. Alternatively, simply delay exercise until blood glucose levels are high enough to start.

Risks for heart disease

Any physical exertion places demands on the heart. While such demands can result in beneficial adaptations, in some people with type 2 diabetes the blood supply to the heart is a limiting factor. In particular, those with heart disease may be limited in their ability to undertake physical exertion. How this occurs is discussed in detail in Chapter 10. Because heart disease is very common in those with type 2 diabetes, before starting any new exercise program all people with diabetes should undergo some assessment of their heart. This may simply mean seeing your doctor, or you might need to undergo an exercise stress test (see earlier in this chapter) to see how the heart copes with physical stress and how safely exercise might be conducted on your own.

Risks for high or low blood pressure

As exercise increases the output of blood from the heart, this can cause an increase in blood pressure levels in some people, especially in those who already have high blood pressure. Rapid rises in blood pressure may lead to heart attacks and strokes and should be avoided where possible in people with type 2 diabetes (see Chapter 10). Such rises can usually be prevented by changing the dose or timing of blood pressure medications. People with uncontrolled hypertension should not begin an exercise program until their blood pressure has been effectively managed.

Some people with type 2 diabetes may also experience a profound fall in blood pressure with exertion. In particular, when diabetes damages the nerves that regulate blood pressure levels, blood pressure levels may be quite brittle and fall significantly with prolonged standing or moderate physical exercise. This may also be seen in some people taking blood pressure-lowering treatments which block the pathways required to keep the blood pressure up. Some doctors will ask you to monitor your blood pressure at home, or carry a continuous monitor for 24 hours (known as **ambulatory blood pressure monitoring**) to look out for falling blood pressure (see Chapter 8).

Risks for foot damage

Diabetes affects circulation to the feet and their ability to sense pain or pressure. This can lead to progressive damage to the feet and is discussed in detail in Chapter 12. Physical exertion can place significant demands on your feet, especially when undertaking activities like walking, running, dancing and other step exercises. Every time your foot strikes the ground it feels the force of nearly twice your body weight.

Everyone with diabetes should undergo regular assessment of their feet anyway. But before starting any new exercise program particular attention should be undertaken to ensure the feet are appropriately protected. For most people this will involve wearing supportive shoes and socks that fit well and do not rub or restrict the circulation. Appropriate shoes should have plenty of room around the forefoot and toes, but be snug enough around the heel to prevent rubbing and blisters. The wrong type of shoe or one that fails to control excessive foot movement can cause pain, blisters or injury.

Good foot hygiene before, during and after exercise is also important. Regularly inspect your feet for damage and change (rather than stop) your physical activity if necessary. It is also useful to consult with a podiatrist regularly, to ensure you haven't missed any early signs of problems and also to keep the nails trimmed, as foot problems with exertion can begin with pressure around sharp nail edges and/or ingrown toenails. A podiatrist can also recommend a specific shoe type or a pair of orthotics to take unwanted pressure off your feet. For people at high risk for foot problems, such as those with insensitive feet or those with previous foot ulcers, more care should be taken in choosing activities that minimise the risk of foot damage — swimming, aquaerobics, cycling, rowing, resistance training, etc. are all good choices.

Support is out there — get help

Exercise is rewarding but it is not easy. In fact, it is supposed to be demanding. This means it can be hard to accomplish and sustain on your own. People generally have greater success with exercise when they have supervision and encouragement from someone else, be that an exercise physiologist, trainer or a local club. Even friends and family can make a real difference in keeping you going strong. There are lots of great programs and resources out there to support you and help you reach your goals. Most of these can be accessed through your diabetes care team and may be subsidised as part of your diabetes care.

Exercise is about doing the right activity in the right doses and at the right pace to achieve your individual goals and needs. No matter what the ads say, there is no generic solution. Different people have different needs, likes and dislikes. Don't be bullied into a gym membership or doing something outside your comfort zone. The exercise program you select needs to become part of your new lifestyle so it must be convenient and enjoyable. When starting out make your exercise program practical, realistic and achievable so that it complements your existing lifestyle without requiring too many changes. When beginning an exercise program after a period of inactivity or unaccustomed exercise, start slowly and stay well within your current capabilities. Set yourself modest but realistic goals, and keep updating them as you get fitter.

It is also important to follow the results of exercise and stay on the right track. Chart the average distances and times of a walking/jogging program and see how you have improved. Keep a record in a diary. Document how weights increase as you undertake your strength program. Watch how your waistline shrinks with a tape measure or changes in your belt size.

Observe the health improvements, like lower blood pressure or cholesterol levels. Enjoy and monitor your progress over time. This can serve as a motivational tool. But, most importantly, it keeps you connected with your exercise and helps you to stay alive.

6

Diabetes pills and injections

UNDERSTAND

» Most people with type 2 diabetes eventually reach a point where some medicines are needed to prevent their glucose levels from rising dangerously.

» Medicines are not an alternative to a good diet and regular exercise, and work better when all are combined.

» There are a number of different medications used to lower glucose levels in people with type 2 diabetes. Each has their benefits as well as the potential for unwanted side effects. Different treatments may be suited to different people and different circumstances.

» The longer you have diabetes, the more likely it will be that insulin may be required. This does not mean you have failed in any way. Type 2 diabetes is a progressive condition in which your ability to make and use insulin declines and ultimately becomes exhausted.

MANAGE

» Learn how your medications work to get the best out of each.

» Make it easier to remember to take your medications by establishing regular routines and using pill packs.

» Coordinate your medications with your diet and lifestyle to ensure the maximum effectiveness of each.

» Discuss with your doctor some of the new options for managing type 2 diabetes and how they might work for you.

A number of different medications are now available to help your body regulate its blood glucose levels. They are not a substitute for a good diet and a regular amount of physical activity. Equally, having to take pills or injections does not mean you're doing something wrong. Most people with type 2 diabetes eventually reach a point where some medicines are needed to prevent their glucose levels from rising dangerously. This is simply the nature of the disease. Over time your pancreas becomes less able to make the insulin it needs to keep glucose levels under control, so it needs more help. The longer you have diabetes, the more likely it will be that you will need one or several different types of medication to keep glucose levels under control. Your doctor will advise which medications may be right for your particular needs. It is important to remember that different treatments may be suited to different people and different circumstances.

This chapter refers to the major classes of medications used to control glucose levels in people with type 2 diabetes and gives the chemical (generic) names of pills and injections rather than their brand names. These chemical names are usually displayed on the packet, under the brand name in smaller writing. There are many different brands and formulations of various products, and these often vary in different countries.

It is important for everyone with type 2 diabetes to know what medications they are taking and how they work to get the most out of them.

If you can't make out or understand the chemical name of your medication and how it fits into this chapter, please consult your doctor, pharmacist or diabetes care team.

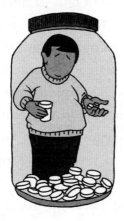

Most people with type 2 diabetes eventually reach a point where some medicines are needed to prevent their glucose levels from rising dangerously. This is simply the nature of the disease.

Metformin

Metformin is the most widely used pill to treat diabetes. Between half and two-thirds of all people with type 2 diabetes take metformin, either alone or in combination with other pills or insulin. It is widely considered to be the first choice of medical treatment to improve glucose control in people with type 2 diabetes. Metformin is thought to have particular advantages for those who are overweight. Recent data have suggested that metformin can also modestly reduce the risk of heart disease, strokes and possibly some cancers, beyond its effects on glucose levels.

Metformin was originally developed from natural compounds found in French lilac (also known as goat's rue or *Galega officinalis*). Extracts from this plant have been used as a traditional treatment of diabetes and other ailments since the Middle Ages. Subsequent studies identified the specific chemicals (known as **biguanides**) that gave it the ability to lower glucose levels. Metformin is the only biguanide used for the treatment of diabetes.

One of the reasons why glucose levels remain elevated in people with type 2 diabetes is that insulin fails to suppress the production of glucose by the liver (see Chapter 1). Consequently, the liver continues to make and secrete large amounts of glucose even when glucose levels are already high. Metformin is able to reduce glucose production by the liver by approximately one-third. However, even with this treatment glucose production by the liver is still elevated in people with type 2 diabetes, on average at least twice that of people without diabetes. Metformin also increases the body's sensitivity to the effects of insulin, improves the uptake of glucose by muscle and slows the absorption of glucose from a meal. When taken as directed, metformin will reduce your HbA1c by approximately 0.5 to 1 per cent.

Unlike with other anti-diabetic medications, low blood glucose levels (hypos) are seldom observed when metformin is used on its own. This is because it does not increase insulin levels or interfere with the body's responses to hypoglycaemia. Metformin also has the advantage over other agents in that it does not cause weight gain and in some people with diabetes it may reduce their weight slightly.

To work effectively most people will need to take 1 to 2 grams of metformin every day. Consequently, metformin tablets will usually be the biggest tablets in size that most people with type 2 diabetes will take. Some people find them difficult to swallow. A metformin syrup formulation taken as drops can be helpful if swallowing the big metformin tablets is a problem for you.

The most commonly reported side effects from metformin include gastrointestinal disturbances (e.g. nausea, diarrhoea, cramping, flatulence). These side effects will affect around one in five people using metformin to some degree but they are usually mild, only seen when using high doses or transiently when first starting metformin. The likelihood of developing side effects can usually be reduced or avoided by taking the following steps:

» Take your metformin with or after meals rather than before meals.

» Your doctor can start you at a low dose, once or twice a day.

» Increase your dose of metformin very gradually (e.g. increase by one pill every fortnight until reaching your target dose).

» Always divide the dose through the day.

» Use extended release (XR) formulations of metformin — these have become preferred for the initial treatment of type 2 diabetes. This is mostly because of the convenience of a once-daily treatment that doesn't need to be coordinated with meals but achieves roughly the same level of glucose control as standard metformin, which you have to take twice or three times a day. The frequency of the gastrointestinal side effects may also be reduced when using XR tablets.

» Do not use too much metformin (in some people). Because metformin is removed from the body by the kidneys, people with type 2 diabetes who are over 70 years old and those with impaired kidney function will require lower doses to maintain safe levels and prevent side effects (e.g. 1 gram per day).

But despite these manoeuvres, about 10 per cent of people with type 2 diabetes are still not able to take metformin because of its side effects.

More seriously, metformin has been associated with an extremely rare but life-threatening condition known as **lactic acidosis**. It is still controversial whether metformin is the instigating cause or whether it exacerbates this condition when it is caused by other things such as heart failure, liver or kidney failure. For this reason, those with heart conditions, a heavy alcohol intake or impaired kidney or liver function should only use metformin with caution and close supervision by their doctor. Metformin should also be temporarily stopped during any major illness (e.g. acute gastroenteritis, heart attack, bone fracture) and prior to major surgery or procedures that might precipitate a sudden fall in kidney function, such as imaging of the arteries using injections of dye (known as contrast angiography). Assuming no problems, metformin can be started again once you have recovered from your procedure.

Sulphonylureas

Sulphonylureas are currently used by about half of all people with type 2 diabetes, mostly in combination with metformin. They are by far the most common 'second-line' agent for treating diabetes after metformin, because of their low cost, their effectiveness in rapidly lowering glucose levels and their long history of use in the treatment of type 2 diabetes.

The anti-diabetic effect of sulphonylureas was discovered quite by accident during World War II, when it was found that some sulphur-containing antibiotics (known as sulphonamides) caused low blood glucose levels in animals. These were then tested in people with type 2 diabetes with outstanding results. Within 10 years sulphonylureas became the first widely used oral medications for the treatment of type 2 diabetes, providing the first real alternative to insulin injections.

A number of different sulphonylureas are currently available. There are many different formulations, brand names and manufacturers. However, in common, the generic name of sulphonylureas usually begins in the prefix 'gli-' including:

- » glipizide
- » gliclazide
- » glibenclamide (also known as glyburide)
- » glibornuride
- » gliquidone
- » glisoxepide
- » glyclopyramide
- » glimepiride.

By and large, they all have comparable actions on glucose levels. However, certain sulphonylureas may be suited to certain clinical situations because of their differing mode of clearance from the body, duration of action and risk of hypoglycaemia.

Sulphonylureas work by triggering the release of insulin from the pancreas, which then works to lower glucose levels as detailed in Chapter 1. Sulphonylureas have the advantage of producing a rapid improvement in glucose control once treatment is initiated. When taken as directed, sulphonylureas will reduce the HbA1c by between 0.5 and 1 per cent in most people with type 2 diabetes. However, this approach also has a number of disadvantages, including:

- » *Hypoglycaemia.* Sulphonylureas can cause low blood glucose levels in some people with type 2 diabetes by stimulating insulin production and release in excess of their requirements, especially if they are missing meals or undertaking unplanned or excessive physical activity. (This is discussed in more detail in Chapter 7.)
- » *Weight gain.* Sulphonylureas can cause modest weight gain (2–3kg/4½–6½lb) in some people. This is mostly seen in the first few months after sulphonylureas are started, and it usually doesn't get worse when treatment is continued. Weight gain is caused by increasing your insulin levels,

whose job it is to get glucose and fat out of the bloodstream, at the expense of increasing your fat deposits.

» *Exhaustion.* Some doctors think that by stimulating the pancreas to make more insulin all the time, without a break, sulphonylureas can progressively burn out the capacity for insulin production over time (known as **beta-cell exhaustion**). This may be one reason why there can sometimes be a gradual loss of glucose control achieved with sulphonylureas with their long-term use over time. In a small number of people (less than 10 per cent) sulphonylureas are completely ineffective in controlling glucose levels when used on their own. This may be because the ability to make insulin is completely exhausted already.

Other uncommon side effects of sulphonylureas include headache, abdominal upset and allergic reactions. Sulphonylureas can sometimes interact with alcohol to produce unpleasant hangover-like symptoms in some people about 10 minutes after drinking and sometimes lasting several hours.

Meglitinides

Meglitinides (known as 'glitinides' or 'glinides') are quick-acting pills that are used to swiftly lower glucose levels after eating. They are taken with the first bite of each meal and rapidly stimulate the release of insulin from the pancreas, through some of the same pathways used by sulphonylureas with which they should not be combined. Glitinides work fast and only for a short time (less than 4 hours). This rapid increase and fall in insulin levels effectively reproduces what happens in healthy people who eat a meal, when insulin levels rapidly rise after each meal and fall as all the food is digested.

There are currently only two different 'glitinides' available, which have in common a chemical (generic) suffix '-glinide':

» repaglinide
» nateglinide.

When taken as directed, glitinides will reduce the HbA1c by 0.5 to 1 per cent in most people with type 2 diabetes. They are very effective in people who have a large rise in glucose levels after meals, but whose glucose control is fine at other times, including during the night.

However, their rapid action can also be a disadvantage as it can quickly cause a rapid drop in glucose levels if not coordinated with a meal (see Chapter 7). This can be partly prevented by only taking the tablets when starting to eat. Yet because of the need to take these tablets three times a day and carefully coordinating them with your meals, glitinides are only sparingly used and generally reserved for selected and fastidious patients. Some people also experience gastrointestinal disturbances (e.g. nausea, abdominal pain, indigestion) with glitinides.

Glitazones

Thiazolidinediones (also known as 'glitazones' or TZDs) were introduced to diabetes care over a decade ago, with much fanfare and great expectations. Glitazones are able to increase the body's sensitivity to the glucose-lowering actions of insulin in muscle and the liver, in a manner different (and complementary) to metformin. When taken as directed, glitazones reduce the HbA1c by 0.5 to 1 per cent in most people with type 2 diabetes. In some people, glitazones are an extremely effective way of controlling blood glucose levels when other drugs are not working. And like metformin, hypoglycaemia is not seen when glitazones are used on their own.

There are currently only two different glitazones available, which have in common a chemical (generic) suffix '-glitazone':

» rosiglitazone
» pioglitazone.

Unfortunately, the risk of serious side effects has limited the use of this glucose-lowering medication. Glitazones can cause fluid retention which leads to weight gain, ankle swelling and even heart failure in susceptible people. Some studies have suggested rosiglitazone may also modestly increase the risk of heart attacks. It is generally recommended that people with type 2 diabetes known to have heart disease should use some other kind of medication to control their blood glucose. Some studies have also suggested glitazones may increase the risk of vision-threatening eye disease and some cancers when compared to other therapies. Glitazones can also thin your bones, which may increase fracture risk in susceptible people, especially older women. Taken together, the side effect profile of glitazones (as opposed to the comparative safety of other classes of medication for treating diabetes) has seen a steady decline in their use in people with diabetes. However, for some people with type 2 diabetes the benefits of glitazones on their glucose control may outweigh the potential for harm.

Incretin agonists

Incretins are natural hormones that amplify the amount of insulin released from the pancreas when eating. This is why they are called incretins (because they **increase** insulin production). Unlike sulphonylureas, they do not stimulate the production of insulin directly. In fact, they only work to boost production when there is another signal to stimulate insulin release, such as food or elevated glucose levels. They don't work when glucose levels are low because insulin production is naturally suppressed. So incretins do not cause hypoglycaemia unless combined with an excess of sulphonylureas or insulin.

While the human body has its own incretins (called GLP-1 and GIP), their effect is not very powerful or long lasting. This is possibly because the human body is best adapted for grazing on carbohydrates (small amounts of food more often) than it is for eating large amounts at once. But this is not true for other animals. For example, in the Sonoran Desert in the United States lives a venomous lizard, the Gila monster. It eats only once every month or two. And when it does, it goes to town, eating up to one-third of its body weight. In the desert you never know when your next meal is coming so you have to make the most of it. But what is most remarkable about this lizard's adaptation to its 'binge eating' lifestyle is that it secretes an incretin into its saliva that has a powerful effect on its metabolism. It is able to remarkably boost insulin release from its pancreas severalfold to allow it to better cope with eating large amounts in one sitting.

This lizard incretin is similar to that found in humans, but subtly different in that it works much better and for longer. And not only for lizards. When injected into humans, a chemical made to look like just like this lizard incretin is also able to amplify insulin release and improve glucose control. It also suppresses appetite and slows the absorption of glucose following a meal, by reducing the rate at which the stomach empties. These two features of incretins also mean that using these injections can bring about weight loss (on average 2–3kg/4½–6½lb).

Although there are a number of incretins currently in clinical development, there are at present only two different injectable incretin agonists available for the treatment of diabetes, which have in common a chemical (generic) suffix '-tide':

» exenatide
» liraglutide.

These are also known as **GLP-agonists** because of their similar mode of action to the human incretin, GLP. Both have comparable actions on glucose levels, reducing the HbA1c by an average of 1 per cent in most patients. Injections may be required twice daily, 1 hour before both breakfast and dinner for shorter acting formulations, to once daily or once weekly for longer acting or slow release forms of these medicines.

Apart from the need to inject, the key disadvantage of these injections is their action on digestion. While slowing the stomach down is a great idea for a venomous lizard that eats once a month, in humans this same effect can upset the stomach in many people. In most cases any discomfort settles gradually over the first month of treatment. When starting off using this kind of medication it is usual to begin with a small dose and then slowly increase the amount you take over a month to limit these side effects. The longer acting formulations (which are generally used in lower doses) cause fewer stomach side effects.

The GLP-1 agonists are among the newest medications used for the treatment of type 2 diabetes. While they certainly work to lower glucose levels, nobody has taken them for more than a few years. Whether they are beneficial or even completely safe in the long term remains to be established.

DPP-4 inhibitors

DPP-4 is an enzyme that breaks down your natural incretin hormones. One of the reasons that the injectable incretins detailed above have such powerful effects on human metabolism is that they are partly resistant to DPP-4, so hang around long enough in high enough levels to get the job done. However, you can achieve the same sort of effect by inhibiting the DPP-4 enzyme that breaks down your own incretins (using pills known as **gliptins**). This means your own incretins can also hang around long enough in high enough levels to get the job done. In essence, instead of bringing the (Gila) monster to you, these pills bring out your own inner monster. These are among the newest drugs available for the treatment of type 2 diabetes.

There are currently only five different DPP-4 inhibitors available for the treatment of diabetes, which have in common a chemical (generic) suffix '-gliptin':

» sitagliptin
» saxagliptin
» linagliptin
» vildagliptin
» allogliptin.

Through inhibiting DPP-4, these pills elevate your natural incretin levels three- to fivefold and thereby further amplify the amount of insulin released from your pancreas after eating or in response to elevated glucose levels. This has roughly the same effect as injecting a GLP-1 agonist, reducing the HbA1c by 0.5 to 1 per cent on average in most people with type 2 diabetes. Gliptins are currently used largely as 'second-line agents' in people already taking metformin, as an alternative to sulphonylureas or insulin, although they are effective on their own as a first-line therapy or combined with TZDs.

The key advantage of gliptins is that they can be taken in tablet form once (or at the most, twice) daily. They can be taken any time of the day, with or without food and do not require coordination with meals or physical activity. Again, this is because they are amplifiers not stimulators of insulin release. They only work when there is a stimulus, such as a meal or having high glucose levels. But if glucose levels are low, there is no signal to make insulin so there is no incretin effect and no risk of hypoglycaemia when used on their own. Gliptins also do not cause weight gain and may bring about weight loss of 1 to 2kg (2¼–4½lb) in some people.

While the gliptins have a number of theoretical advantages, this class of medication is still quite new. This means that they are more costly, and therefore tend to be restricted in their use when compared to other treatments that have been around for many decades. Again, whether they are beneficial or even completely safe in the long term remains to be established.

Acarbose

Acarbose is a natural product derived from cultured bacteria. Most of the glucose you get from your diet comes from the digestion of starch contained in carbohydrate-rich food. Acarbose temporarily blocks the enzymes that digest starch, meaning that instead of being broken down immediately and entering the body, it takes much longer for glucose to get into the body from each meal. This effect is much like converting a high GI meal into a low GI meal. This slower rate of absorption better matches the limited rate of insulin secretion typical in people with type 2 diabetes. Since it only works briefly, acarbose is taken three times a day at the start of each meal.

Although acarbose modestly lowers blood glucose levels, it does not cause hypoglycaemia when taken on its own as it does not interfere with the body's ability to make glucose. However, if someone is having a hypo due to other anti-diabetic medications they are also taking, acarbose can prevent consumed starchy foods from raising glucose levels and treat the hypo. Consequently, if someone taking acarbose is having a hypo they must eat pre-digested sugars such as glucose tablets or fruit juice, rather than starchy foods, to reverse the fall in glucose levels.

But while preventing the digestion of carbohydrates, acarbose allows more starch to reach the lower parts of the intestine, where it is happily digested by bacteria. This releases gas, and sometimes lots of it. This will cause significant flatulence in most people and result in bloating, discomfort or diarrhoea in others. These side effects can usually be reduced by starting at a lower dose (25mg once a day) and gradually increasing over a month (to 100mg three times a day). Symptoms will generally settle after a month or two of regular use. However, some people will not be able to tolerate these effects at all. As a result, acarbose is not widely used in the management of type 2 diabetes outside of developing countries.

Some studies have suggested that acarbose reduces the risk of colon cancer, partly through nourishing your healthy gut bacteria. Acarbose may also have other useful effects on clotting, blood pressure and lipid levels. This has been suggested as one reason it appears to modestly reduce the risk of heart attacks and strokes in those with diabetes, over and above its effect on lowering glucose levels.

SGLT2 inhibition

Another way to reduce an excess amount of glucose in the bloodstream is to allow it to pass harmlessly into your urine. This is exactly what normally happens when glucose levels are too high — it spills over into the urine. This is the reason why people with diabetes may pass large amounts of slightly sweet urine (hence the term 'diabetes mellitus' which means 'siphon of honey'). However, it is possible to further enhance the loss of glucose into the urine by blocking the pathways that would normally retrieve it from the urine and prevent the valuable energy source from being lost.

It has been known for some time that the bark of pear, apple, cherry and other fruit trees contains a bitter-tasting chemical that causes glucose to be lost into the urine. This compound also inhibits the absorption of glucose from the intestine. More recently, companies have developed more selective chemicals that only block the kidney pathways. These drugs (known as **SGLT2 inhibitors**) have just recently become available for the management of type 2 diabetes.

There are currently three different SGLT2 inhibitors available for the treatment of diabetes, which have in common a chemical (generic) suffix '-gliflozin':

» dapagliflozin

» canagliflozin

» empagliflozin.

When used as directed, these agents lower HbA1c levels by 0.5 to 1 per cent. Because they have no effect on insulin release they do not cause hypoglycaemia, and glucose will not spill into the urine if blood glucose levels are low anyway. By losing the excess calories contained in glucose, this treatment may also be associated with some weight loss (1–2kg/2¼–4½lb) and reductions in blood pressure.

However, having glucose in your urine has its downside too. It means passing more urine more frequently, which can be an issue in those with a troublesome bladder. It can also increase the risk of bladder and genital infections, although these are typically mild and easily managed when you are on the lookout for them. Long-term studies are yet to be completed.

Insulin

Insulin is the most important regulator of blood glucose levels in the human body. If glucose levels are too high, then insulin is not doing its job. For nearly a century it has been recognised that injecting insulin can reduce glucose levels and maintain glucose control in people with type 2 diabetes.

All people with type 1 diabetes must take insulin due to irreversible damage to the insulin-producing cells of their pancreas.

In some people with type 2 diabetes, the different medications that assist in the release of insulin or its actions are not enough to maintain glucose control. If this happens your doctor may consider starting insulin.

This does not mean you have failed in any way. Type 2 diabetes is a progressive condition in which your ability to make and use insulin declines and ultimately becomes exhausted. The longer you have diabetes, the more likely it will be that insulin may be required.

Injecting insulin is the most effective way to lower your glucose levels. When taken as directed, insulin injections will reduce the HbA1c by 1 to 2 per cent in most people with type 2 diabetes. The insulin injection works in the same way as the insulin made naturally in your pancreas — it stimulates the removal of glucose from the bloodstream and its storage in the tissues of your body, as well as stopping the liver making more glucose.

Insulin is injected into the fat under the skin (known as a subcutaneous injection). The best place is usually the fatty areas on your abdomen or thighs. You might think injections are difficult, painful or embarrassing, but it is actually quite easy to become proficient. The needles used to inject the insulin are very small. Most people say the injections are less painful than pricking the finger to test blood glucose levels. Most insulin syringes are very discreet. Many are indistinguishable from large fountain pens with a cartridge of insulin inserted like an ink cartridge. These make insulin injections quite straightforward since drawing up the medicine into the syringe is unnecessary. You just need to dial up the dose you want to use and inject.

There are many different insulin formulations that vary in how rapidly they deliver insulin and how long they continue to provide it. These will suit different people and situations. The most common varieties include:

» **rapid-acting insulin** which is injected immediately before meals, one to three times a day
» **intermediate** and **long-acting insulin** (also known as **basal insulin**) which is injected once a day, usually at bedtime or breakfast
» a mix of short- and long-acting insulins (known as **pre-mix insulin**) which is usually injected twice a day.

It is common to start out insulin injections for someone with type 2 diabetes with a low dose (8–10 units) of intermediate or long-acting insulin at bedtime or once in the morning (for those who have high glucose levels during the day). This is then slowly adjusted in small increments (e.g. 2–4 units every 2–4 days) as required to get control of glucose levels. The final dose usually ends up being between 20 and 40 units a day but can vary considerably between different people. This period of adjustment is quite intensive and always requires frequent contact with your diabetes team. You will generally also need to keep taking some or all of your oral anti-diabetic medications, to help the injected insulin to work effectively.

Because insulin is able to lower your glucose levels, no matter what level they are, blood glucose levels can sometimes fall to very low levels in people using insulin injections and cause a hypo (see Chapter 7). But even then it is not very common to have hypos. Hypos may be more likely when you are starting out, when the right dose and timing are first being assessed. This is also why the slow supervised start to insulin detailed above is so important. The chance of having a hypo is also increased in people who don't take their medications regularly, and those whose diet or lifestyle are irregular (different levels of physical activity, different amounts and types of food, skipping meals, etc.). But while hypos can sound scary, most can be prevented by good diabetes management.

Starting insulin is also often associated with increased appetite and unwanted weight gain (often between 2–5kg/ 4½–11lb). This occurs because insulin's main job is to drive glucose out of the blood by making and storing fat. Some new specially modified forms of insulin seem to cause less weight gain while achieving the same or better glucose control.

Complementary therapies

All of the medicines detailed in this chapter are backed by scientific evidence that demonstrates their effectiveness in people with diabetes. However, there are also many other products that are marketed for those with type 2 diabetes to improve your glucose control. You will see them every day in the pharmacy, in the supermarket or on the internet. It is appealing to think that they may help you to better manage your glucose levels. However, none of these should be considered 'alternative medicines' for the management of diabetes. In fact, there is evidence of significant health risks when such remedies replace standard-of-care treatment.

The most widely sold supplements for diabetes contain

trace elements, including chromium, zinc, magnesium and/or vanadium. But while each of these minerals has been reported to have effects on glucose levels in some studies, this has not been borne out in other studies and larger trials. At best the effects are very modest, lowering the HbA1c by less than 0.3 per cent.

Plants and their extracts have been used in traditional (folk) medicine for the treatment of diabetes for thousands of years. In fact, the most widely used medicine for lowering glucose levels, metformin, was originally derived from a traditional diabetes remedy. While a number of different herbs have been shown to lower glucose levels in some people, their effects are small at best and quite variable. They will not work in the majority of patients (unlike known diabetes medications). The long-term effectiveness and the potential for serious side effects of many of these herbs remain to be clarified. At present there is no evidence to recommend their use in people with type 2 diabetes.

Some herbs reported to have glucose-lowering effects include:

- » American ginseng (*Panax. quiquefolius*)
- » aloe vera
- » bitter melon (*Momordica charantia*)
- » cinnamon (*Cinnamomum verum*)
- » ivy gourd (*Coccinia indica*)
- » fenugreek (*Trigonella foenum-graecum*)
- » garlic (*Allium sativum*)
- » holy basil (*Ocimum sanctum*)
- » gurmar (*Gymnema sylvestre*)
- » nopal or prickly pear cactus (*Opuntia streptacantha*)
- » huang lian (*Rhizoma coptidis*)
- » Russian tarragon (*Artemisia dracunculus*).

7.
Swing low

UNDERSTAND

» The brain requires a constant supply of glucose to function. If glucose levels fall below 3mmol/L (54mg/dL), then the brain's functions can become impaired.

» Most people with type 2 diabetes have little or no risk of having a hypo.

» Some of the medicines that lower glucose levels in people with type 2 diabetes have the potential to cause hypoglycaemia under certain circumstances. The most common reason for a hypo is that there is too much insulin for your prevailing glucose level.

» In the minority of people with type 2 diabetes who experience a hypo, changes to their lifestyle and medications can significantly reduce the risk of further episodes.

MANAGE

» Talk to your doctor about your risks for having a hypo, based on the type of medication you are using and the targets for your treatment.

» If you are at risk, develop and execute an action plan of what you would do in the event of a hypo. Always be prepared.

» If you suspect a hypo, get on and treat it, since the risks of failing to treat a hypo outweigh those of unnecessary treatment.

» Take special precautions to make sure you don't 'swing low' when driving.

» Limit the amount of alcohol you drink and always combine alcohol with food.

The brain needs a continuous supply of glucose to function. And not just a little. Over half of all glucose made by the body is subsequently used by the brain. For the brain, glucose in the blood is just as important as the oxygen in the air you breathe. The brain cannot last more than a few minutes without it. The brain can't make its own glucose. Instead, it requires a continuous supply of glucose in the bloodstream to keep it going.

It's easy to keep your glucose levels up while you are eating. But you can't eat all the time. And when you're not eating, the body must still maintain roughly the same glucose levels as always. To achieve this, a healthy pancreas directs a coordinated response to keep your glucose levels steady. This response includes:

» stimulating the synthesis and release of new glucose from the liver

» releasing fat from its stores, which is then used as an alternative fuel source by most organs (except the brain) — this effectively spares glucose for exclusive use by your brain

» suppressing the release of insulin, whose job it is to lower glucose levels and put fat back into storage — this is the opposite of what is needed when glucose levels are already low.

Consequently, dangerously low glucose levels cannot occur in healthy people, even in those who undertake prolonged fasting or fad diets that are very low in energy. Your metabolism is programmed to look after your brain and its best interests.

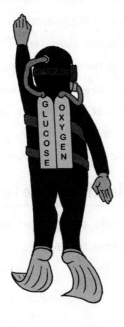

For the brain, glucose is just as important as the oxygen in the air you breathe. The brain cannot last for more than a few minutes without either.

Most people with type 2 diabetes have too little insulin and their body makes too much glucose (see Chapter 1). This is why their glucose levels are generally too high. Consequently, in people with type 2 diabetes who are not on any glucose-lowering medications there is little or no risk that glucose levels will fall too low (known as **hypoglycaemia**).

Diabetes does not cause hypoglycaemia. Hypoglycaemia can only occur if one or all of these protective mechanisms fails to kick in when glucose levels are falling.

The most likely trigger is that there is too much insulin present when glucose levels are already low. This can sometimes occur in people with type 2 diabetes if they are also taking medications that increase their insulin levels (sulphonylureas and meglitinides) or are injecting insulin itself. The other medications used to treat diabetes cannot increase insulin levels when glucose is low, so can't cause hypoglycaemia on their own.

Hypoglycaemia can also occur in people with type 2 diabetes if glucose production by the liver is suppressed when it should be turned on full to keep your glucose levels up. This may occur in those taking glucose-lowering medications who also drink too much alcohol or drink alcohol on an empty stomach. Alcohol suppresses the production of glucose by the liver. So if levels are already swinging low with your medication, they are likely to swing lower and swing faster if you have also been drinking.

What happens when glucose levels fall too low?

To protect against low glucose levels, the human body triggers a number of 'early warning' symptoms including:

» hunger
» looking pale
» sweating
» palpitations (pounding heartbeat)
» increased pulse rate
» tingling sensation (known as parathesia), often around the lips
» shaking/trembling
» headache
» nausea.

These symptoms are collectively experienced as what is commonly termed a **hypo**. The severity of these symptoms partly depends on how low the glucose levels go and how rapidly they fall. Generally, the body's warning symptoms first kick in as glucose falls below 3.5mmol/L (63mg/dL). However, some people can experience no warning signs until glucose levels fall to lower levels. For example, older people with type 2 diabetes generally experience warning signals for a hypo at lower glucose levels than in younger people.

At least initially, these warning symptoms of hypoglycaemia may be mild and readily ignored, especially if your mind is focused on other matters. Many of these symptoms might also occur for reasons other than hypoglycaemia in people with type 2 diabetes. For example, low blood pressure has very similar effects on the body and the brain when compared to those caused by low glucose levels. However, if it is a hypo, all these symptoms will be rapidly improved by taking sweet food or drinks, making it usually possible to quickly distinguish low glucose levels from other causes of illness.

Not all people will experience the same warning signs with a hypo, which are often unique to any given person. For the minority of people with type 2 diabetes who experience hypos as a result of their treatment, it is important for them to become familiar with their own signals that tell them their glucose levels are low and the scenarios in which they occur, and use them to recognise that it is time to do something about them (see 'How do you treat hypoglycaemia?' later in this chapter).

If these early warning symptoms pass unheeded and glucose levels drop further, the brain becomes starved of the glucose (energy) it needs, and all of its functions begin to slow down. This can lead to:

» faintness

» drowsiness

» loss of attention/concentration/performance

» delayed reflexes

» confusion/impaired judgement

» anxiety/moodiness/shakiness

» blurred vision

» disturbed sleep/nightmares

» slurred speech

» unsteadiness.

Rarely is a hypo so incapacitating to the brain that you need the assistance of others to get right again. It is very unusual to completely lose consciousness. But it is hard to do the simple things you need to do to fix low glucose levels if your brain is starved of the glucose it needs to work properly. And this means you may need help. For the minority of people who suffer lots of hypos, carrying or wearing some form of identification that clearly states you have diabetes and you are on medication that can cause hypos may be appropriate.

These symptoms of brain 'slow down' are not generally seen unless glucose levels fall below 3mmol/L (54mg/dL). But some people with diabetes may experience this slow down at higher glucose levels, especially if glucose levels have been falling rapidly. This is why it is better to treat a suspected hypo than to wait and see what the glucose level is.

However, one of the biggest problems about hypos is the lengths some people feel they need to go to in order to avoid them. Hypos are scary. Anyone who has experienced one knows how upsetting they are, and how important it is that you do everything in your power to prevent them from occurring again. Consequently, the fear of hypoglycaemia is one of the most important barriers to good glucose control and is a key reason why current treatments cannot achieve the level of glucose control seen in people without diabetes. For example, hypos can be a major reason to compromise your glucose control and accept values where the risk of hypoglycaemia might be lower.

Sometimes the fear of hypoglycaemia can also restrict the things you feel you can do, including exercise or social activities. But it does not have to be this way. As discussed in the previous chapter there are now many new medications for managing diabetes that don't increase the risk of hypoglycaemia. So rather than compromise, it is possible to tailor the right medications for the right patients.

What triggers a hypo?

As detailed above, hypos can occur in people with type 2 diabetes if they are also taking medications that increase their insulin levels (sulphonylureas and meglitinides) or are injecting insulin itself. However, even here the risk of hypos is low, and the majority of people taking these medicines do not ever experience hypos. That said, hypos may sometimes occur in the following circumstances:

» If you take too much (dose) of these medications.

» If you take these medications at the wrong time or wrong time interval.

» If you accumulate too much of these medicines in your system (as may occur in people with kidney disease).

» If your medicines are acting too quickly, such as when accidentally injecting insulin into muscle (instead of fat) which can also sometimes lead to faster absorption of insulin and drop glucose levels faster than planned.

» If your medicines start working better. As your health improves with good diabetes management, it is common for your medications to get better at lowering your glucose levels. In fact, it is quite common to become more 'sensitive' to the actions of insulin. This is one of the key benefits of good diabetes control. However, when insulin works better, some people find that the high doses of the medications they needed before may become too high, and some dose reduction is required in order to prevent hypoglycaemia. Even when taking the right medications, at the right time and in the right doses, it is also possible to drop glucose levels too much by failing to coordinate diabetes management with your lifestyle. Some common precipitants of a hypo involve irregular or changing lifestyle circumstances, such as missing or delaying a meal or meals, or radically changing your diet (e.g. eating meals that contain less carbohydrate than usual).

It is a common misconception that those with diabetes need to snack regularly between meals to avoid hypos.

This is usually unnecessary and is an important source of unwanted calories and weight gain. Many so-called 'snacks' provide as many calories as a normal meal. Certainly, in those people prone to hypos, having healthy snacks available can be useful in the event of unforeseen activity or changes in the timing or amount of meals. But overeating to prevent hypoglycaemia is never a solution.

Excessive physical activity (commonly more prolonged or more vigorous than what you are used to) may sometimes also trigger a hypo in those who can't buffer falling glucose levels because of their treatment.

Blood glucose is normally used up by any physical activity, and at a greater rate during vigorous exercise. This is why it is so effective in controlling glucose levels in type 2 diabetes. But it is also why it can sometimes lead to hypos in some circumstances.

Exercise not only uses up glucose, it can also slow the emptying of food from the stomach so that sugars from food may be delivered more slowly than expected. Exercise also slows down the body's ability to make and release glucose, so low glucose levels may still occur many hours after physical activity.

The solution is not to avoid exercise. The majority of people with type 2 diabetes have glucose levels that are high enough to buffer the effects of exercise and never get close to significant lows. For the minority who do experience hypos with exercise, they can be prevented by better coordinating physical activity and medication. For example, don't exercise straight after taking your medication. Another solution may be to eat a carbohydrate-rich snack if blood glucose levels are less than 5.5mmol/L (100mg/dL) before starting your exercise.

The stress of being unwell, for whatever reason, changes the amount of insulin your body needs. It also often changes the amount and type of food you eat. Under these circumstances it is common for glucose control to get out of hand, with more highs but also sometimes a greater risk for hypos. If you become unwell it is important to alert your diabetes team early, so that your medications can be adjusted accordingly.

As mentioned earlier in this chapter, drinking too much alcohol or drinking alcohol on an empty stomach can suppress the production of glucose by the liver. This is an essential buffer for low glucose levels, so alcohol increases the risk and severity of hypoglycaemia. If you are intoxicated it may also be hard for you (or anyone else) to recognise you are low and start treatment in a timely fashion. Having diabetes does not mean you have to give up drinking. However, moderation is important in people with diabetes, especially those who experience hypos. In addition, always remembering to eat some carbohydrate-rich food when you are drinking can be a helpful safeguard against falling glucose levels. (See pp. 156–157 for recommended alcohol amounts.)

Diabetes and driving

There are some other circumstances where special preventive management for hypoglycaemia is also appropriate. One of the most important is when planning to drive a car, particularly on long journeys.

Most people with type 2 diabetes are healthy and are able to drive without restrictions. Some countries have specific restrictions on your fitness to drive that prevent you driving a car if you have a high risk of hypoglycaemia. Other countries allow you to drive only after a medical certificate has been received and this may need to be updated every few years depending on the medication you are using and the presence of other complications, including eye problems and heart disease.

If you have experienced a hypo, you'll know it's not something you'd want to happen while you are driving. So for those people with type 2 diabetes who are at risk for hypos there are some simple precautions you can take before and while driving to minimise your risks and keep you and others safe:

» Have a meal before setting out on a long journey.
» Check your glucose levels before driving and every 2 hours while driving.
» Never get behind the wheel if you have low blood glucose levels or are experiencing symptoms, even if it is not far to home.
» Be proactive about treating falling levels — don't wait until you feel symptoms.
» Although snacking all the time can be a problem, having a supply of snacks which you can safely and easily reach while driving is a good precaution for a long journey.
» Never drink and drive, as alcohol makes hypos more likely and more severe.

How do you treat hypoglycaemia?

You should always intervene if you experience symptoms suggestive of a hypo. Measuring your blood glucose level first can be informative. It will usually be less than 3.5mmol/L (63mg/dL). But if you suspect a hypo it is better to treat it immediately, since the risks of not treating a hypo outweigh the risks associated with unnecessary treatment.

If you are having a hypo, immediately take any one of the suggestions below:

20g of glucose (tablets, powder or five to seven jelly beans, depending on their size)

1 tablespoon of jam/honey or table sugar

half a glass of fruit juice or a regular soft drink (not 'diet' drinks).

If symptoms persist, repeat the dose in 10 minutes. When your symptoms have resolved, give the glucose another 10 minutes to be fully absorbed, then eat a carbohydrate-rich snack (e.g. a piece of fruit, glass of milk, a tub of yoghurt, six small dry biscuits or a sandwich), or if your next main meal is nearly due then just start early.

This should then be followed up with your diabetes care team so that changes can be made where necessary to your medication, diet or physical activity. In most cases repeat episodes can be prevented without having to rely on treatment to save the day all the time.

8.
Under pressure

UNDERSTAND

» The level of blood pressure that represents hypertension has been broadly defined as a systolic blood pressure of 140mmHg or higher or a diastolic blood pressure 90mmHg or higher.

» Hypertension is at least twice as common in people who have type 2 diabetes as in those who do not have diabetes.

» High blood pressure is an important cause of complications in people with type 2 diabetes. For every 1mmHg increase in the systolic blood pressure, the long-term risk of heart attack or stroke will increase by 2 to 3 per cent.

» Most people with type 2 diabetes need medications (known as anti-hypertensives) to control their blood pressure levels and reduce their risk of complications.

» Diet and lifestyle changes can not only lower blood pressure levels but also reduce the need for medication(s) and improve their effectiveness.

MANAGE

» Get your blood pressure checked every time you see your doctor, even if you don't have high blood pressure or are not receiving medication.

» Obtain an accurate assessment of what your blood pressure is really doing over the course of your day with ambulatory monitoring, and use it to target and achieve comprehensive blood pressure control.

» Lose that waist. For every 1kg (2¼lb) of weight you lose, your systolic blood pressure will go down on average by approximately 1mmHg.

» Recognise the stress you may be under, and get some assistance in managing it. Find time to relax and make constructive lifestyle changes that help prevent stress.

» Take your medication. A common reason for high blood pressure is non-compliance. Drugs don't work unless you take them.

High blood pressure (hypertension) is an important cause of complications in people with type 2 diabetes. Heart disease, strokes, poor circulation to the legs, eye and kidney damage are more common in people with high blood pressure than in people whose blood pressure is under control. This is partly because high blood pressure causes wear and tear on the walls of the major blood vessels that supply these parts of the body. Its mechanical effects can be likened to the effects of traffic on a road — the greater the pounding of the traffic, the more heavy trucks that roar along its surface, the more likely it is that potholes will occur and that accidents will happen. This is the same for blood pressure, except the accidents are called heart attacks and strokes.

High blood pressure has similar effects on the heart. Literally, the heart is put under pressure. This means it has to work harder to move all the blood around the body, just as it gets harder to put air into a balloon as the pressure inside it increases. In the short term, this extra work causes the heart to grow larger in an attempt to cope with this extra load. However, these extra demands come at some cost. Bigger hearts are also more vulnerable to the effects of poor circulation, such as occurs in type 2 diabetes.

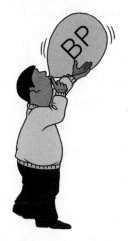

Hypertension means you have increased tension in the walls of your blood vessels, which feel the strain just like a balloon that has been overinflated.

Yet high blood pressure can be prevented and/or treated. Lowering blood pressure will lower the stress on the surface of your heart and blood vessels, just like preventing the passage of heavy trucks will protect a road. In fact, sustained control of blood pressure is one of the most important ways to protect your heart, brain and other organs.

What is blood pressure?

In order to move all your blood around your body once every 4 minutes, your blood must flow fast and never stop. The force of the flowing blood is known as the **blood pressure**. This pressure is not insubstantial (as anyone who has cut themselves accidentally or seen too many horror movies will easily appreciate). However, the pressure of blood is kept in check by the **tension** in the elastic walls of your blood vessels. A similar tension can actually be seen in the walls of a balloon that has been fully inflated, where its 'elastic recoil' resists the expanding pressure of the air so that the balloon stays roughly the same size.

The highest pressure in any blood vessel is generated by the force of contraction of your heartbeat (known as **systole**). This pressure peak is known as the **systolic blood pressure** and is what you feel as your pulse. Systolic blood pressure can be simply measured by using a pressurised cuff to block off the circulation in the arm. When the cuff pressure is higher than the systolic blood pressure, no blood will flow into your arm, which is why it tingles. But as the pressure in the cuff is lowered, there comes a point at which the blood begins to flow again, when the pressure in the cuff is overcome by the force of your heartbeat. This is the systolic blood pressure and is usually between 120 and 140 mmHg.

The lowest pressure in a blood vessel is known as the **diastolic blood pressure**, as it corresponds to the point (known as **diastole**) at which the heart is relaxed and busy filling in order to get ready for its next contraction. Diastolic pressure is usually around 70 to 80mmHg when measured using a blood pressure cuff.

When recording the blood pressure, it is common to report the systolic over the diastolic blood pressure, so that '130 over 80' means a systolic blood pressure of 130mmHg and a diastolic pressure of 80mmHg. The difference between systolic and diastolic pressures is called the **pulse pressure**, as this is a measure of how forceful your pulse seems to be when it is felt at your wrist.

The pressure inside your blood vessels is determined by a number of different factors including:

» *The volume of blood.* Just like air in a balloon, the more air the more pressure. In the same way if there is more fluid retained in the body, for the same space, the pressure in your arteries can increase. Similarly, when people lose large amounts of blood, such as after surgery or following an accident, their blood pressure is also often low.

» *The strength of each heartbeat.* During each contraction of the heart, a small volume of blood is squeezed out. The stronger the heart squeezes, the higher the pressure it is able to generate. Equally, if the heart is not pumping well, the blood pressure can be low, such as in some people with heart failure (see Chapter 10).

» *The elastic recoil of the blood vessels.* Blood vessels have strong elastic walls. These distend in response to the increase in pressure associated with each pulse of pressure generated by your heart. You can sometimes actually see this bulging as the pulse passes through blood vessels in your neck or arms. This stretching is very important as it provides the energy that will help maintain blood pressure after the pulse has passed. This is because after being stretched out by the pulse, the elastic rebound/recoil of the arteries then creates an inward pressure. This serves to maintain blood pressure and therefore a continuous flow of blood until the next contraction of the heart.

One of the best known changes in the blood vessels of people with type 2 diabetes is known as **hardening of the arteries**. This literally means that blood vessels are less compliant or less able to distend. So when each pulse comes along in a hard artery, the systolic pressure will be higher, as instead of distending like a balloon the increased volume with each pulse has nowhere to go. However, diastolic pressure does not tend to rise in hardened arteries, as less distension also means less recoil. This means that hardening of the arteries usually causes an **isolated elevation in systolic blood pressure**, which is the most common change in the blood pressure of adults with type 2 diabetes.

» *The resistance to flow.* Pushing fluid down a large pipe is much easier than pushing the same amount of fluid down a series of small tubes. What makes it hard is known as **resistance**. The higher the resistance to flow, the higher the pressure needed to overcome it. Resistance in your blood vessels is determined in part by the changing diameter of small blood vessels in your circulation (known as **resistance vessels**). If these vessels constrict, the blood pressure goes up as there is more resistance to the flow of blood. To keep flow constant it takes more pressure to overcome more resistance. By contrast, when resistance vessels dilate, the pressure needed to make the blood flow is reduced. Many medications that lower blood pressure chiefly work by dilating resistance vessels (known as vasodilators).

Because high blood pressure is damaging to blood vessels, and low blood pressure is not good either (as it means less blood supply and the oxygen and nutrients it contains), the human body contains a number of mechanisms that keep the blood pressure levels within relatively narrow confines. These sense when the blood pressure is falling, and activate pathways to increase the output from the heart, retain fluid and constrict blood vessels supplying non-essential organs to prop up the blood pressure. Equally, if blood pressure rises, the pathways to dilate blood vessels, remove fluid and restrict the heart's functions become active.

Even so, blood pressure doesn't stay absolutely the same all the time but varies slightly depending on a number of factors:

» *Position.* Blood pressure is usually a little lower when standing up than when sitting or lying down. This is because blood pools in the legs when standing, so less blood gets back to the heart and the pump pressure falls. However, this drop is usually very small because it immediately triggers a reflex response to cause the constriction of resistance blood vessels, and an increase in the heart rate. In some people with type 2 diabetes, their systolic blood pressure can drop very significantly when they stand (more than 20mmHg). This is known as **postural** or **orthostatic hypotension** and in some cases is experienced as dizzy spells or fainting. This drop in blood pressure on standing may be because some medications and/or diabetes itself can interfere with the reflexes required to keep the blood pressure up. Dizziness on standing may also be experienced by people who are dehydrated, anaemic or hot, because such reflexes are already fully active and can't increase further.

» *Sleep.* Systolic blood pressure is generally 10 to 20 per cent lower during sleep when compared to daytime levels. This is known as **nocturnal dipping**. People who don't experience a nightly fall in blood pressure of at least 10 per cent (known as **non-dippers**) have higher rates of complications from their diabetes. Whether this is because blood pressure is not falling at night or because non-dippers have other problems with their blood pressure control is unclear. Nonetheless, some doctors advocate their patients take their blood pressure medication in the evening so that its greatest effect may be at night and first thing in the morning.

» *Stress.* In the short term, blood pressure levels are sometimes higher if you're excited, stressed or nervous.

This is because blood pressure is controlled by the **sympathetic nervous system** (also known as the **fight or flight response**). When you are nervous or stressed, activation of the sympathetic nervous system makes your heart race and beat more strongly, while the resistance vessels constrict. This can sometimes lead to a surge in blood pressure. For example, the blood pressure when seeing your doctor is usually 5 to 10mmHg higher than it is when you are at home. This can sometimes make it appear to your doctor that you have increased blood pressure, even if you don't usually have it at other times (known as white-coat hypertension). However, there is good evidence that any surges in blood pressure may be very important for your health and wellbeing.

» *Mornings.* First thing in the morning, there is normally a surge in blood pressure of between 20 and 30mmHg associated with waking up, rising and becoming physically active after a night's sleep. This increase may be exaggerated in some people and may be one reason why the risk of heart attacks and strokes is greatest in the two hours after getting up in the morning.

» *Exercise.* Although regular exercise can lower blood pressure levels over weeks or months of application, any physical activity can cause a rapid rise in blood pressure in some people. This is why your doctor will usually take your blood pressure after at least 5 minutes of rest. This is also why, before starting an exercise program, a careful assessment of risk should be performed (see Chapter 5). Sometimes doctors counsel some people with diabetes to limit activity because of these concerns, especially those with poorly controlled blood pressure.

» *Food.* Different food or drink in your diet can impact on the development and progression of high blood pressure over the long term. This is discussed in detail below. However, sometimes a meal can also affect blood pressure levels. This is because, when you eat, extra blood is diverted to your intestines to help absorb its nutrients. This can result in a small but significant drop in blood pressure after meals in some people.

» *Gender.* Blood pressure levels are generally higher in men than in women. However, following the menopause this difference is reversed as blood pressure levels rise more rapidly when the protective effects of sex hormones on the blood vessels decline.

How is blood pressure measured?

People with type 2 diabetes should have their blood pressure checked every time they see their doctor, even if they don't have high blood pressure or are not receiving blood pressure medication.

Blood pressure measurements are usually taken when sitting, but measurements taken while standing are also worthwhile to check for the development of postural hypotension. This should be done at least annually or more often if you are experiencing symptoms like dizziness when standing abruptly, or if you have other signs to suggest diabetes has damaged your nerves (e.g. numbness, feet problems, etc.). Blood pressure will sometimes also be measured in both arms to look for differences between the arms that could indicate narrowing of the arteries.

Measuring your blood pressure is usually performed by wrapping an inflatable cuff with a pressure gauge around your arm or wrist. This should fit snugly. If a cuff is too small, it will underestimate your blood pressure. Equally, if the cuff is too large it will produce a higher blood pressure reading than your true blood pressure. Different cuff sizes are available to accommodate for larger or smaller arms and ensure accurate readings.

The pressure in the cuff is then slowly increased until blood flow in the arm is temporarily prevented. In most people this is completely painless. However, some people experience unpleasant numbness or tingling when the cuff is maximally inflated. But it is only for a moment and subsides when the cuff is deflated. It will not cause damage to the arm. Air is then slowly released from the cuff. The point at which blood flow returns to the arm (the systolic blood pressure) can be gauged either by feeling or listening for the pulse. Normally, smooth flow through blood vessels makes no sound. But when the blood first returns to the arm after the cuff is slowly released, with each turbulent spurt of blood that comes down the artery a tapping noise can be heard with a stethoscope, in time with the pulse. When the pressure in the cuff falls below the diastolic pressure, the continuous flow to the arm is fully restored and the sounds of intermittent turbulent flow in blood vessels can no longer be heard; so diastolic pressure is gauged by the sound of silence. For this reason it is harder to measure accurately, especially in noisy environments such as medical practices or shopping malls.

Automated machines that inflate and deflate by themselves are also widely used. In these machines, a sensor (known as an **oscillometer**) is used to detect the return of blood flow to the arm. This can make it easier to detect changes in blood flow without needing to hear it. When standardised and used regularly, such machines are very valuable and are widely used in hospitals and medical clinics. Home oscillometers are also available. Results can vary significantly from machine to machine, but they are generally pretty reliable once standardised and calibrated. So if you have one, take it with you for your next check-up and compare its reading with that taken by your nurse or doctor to make sure they are close to one another. Using the same machine all the time is the best way to ensure that any changes measured in your blood pressure are real.

Ambulatory blood pressure monitoring is emerging as the best way to establish a diagnosis of high blood pressure and to determine the response to treatment in people with type 2 diabetes. Although the word 'ambulatory' makes you think that it means monitoring while you are walking (ambling), in fact this kind of monitoring means taking an automated blood pressure reading every 20 to 30 minutes while you are awake and every 30 to 60 minutes while you are sleeping. This gives a much more accurate picture of what blood pressure levels are over the course of 24 hours. It can detect any surges in blood pressure or any dipping at night or other times. Your blood pressure readings can also be matched with a diary noting what you were doing at the time, or how you felt. The average value of measurements taken during waking hours is often used to confirm a diagnosis of high blood pressure.

Although it might seem cumbersome to carry around a blood pressure device for a day and a night, the machines are surprisingly small and quiet. But the cuff still has to blow up; the most common complaint is that this disturbs your sleep, or that of your bed partner. But it is only for one night.

Home blood pressure monitoring is another way to confirm a diagnosis of high blood pressure. Home monitoring simply means taking your blood pressure twice a day for a week. The average value of all the measurements (ignoring the first day, which is usually higher as you are getting used to the plan) can be used to confirm a diagnosis of high blood pressure. The home monitoring method takes some application, but many people find it better as it does not mean blood pressure measurements through the night. However, this is also its downside, as it does not give information about what is happening at night. Nonetheless, it is still better than basing treatment decisions on just the blood pressure measurements taken when you go to the doctor.

How high is high — what is hypertension?

All pressure applied to blood vessels causes some tension in their walls. This tension progressively leads to changes, or damage, in the way they function. The greater the blood pressure, the greater that damage. The point at which the risk of blood vessel damage is significantly increased is known as **hypertension**. This literally means you have increased tension in the walls of your blood vessels that feel the strain, just like the wall of a balloon that has been overinflated.

The level of blood pressure that represents hypertension is broadly defined as:

» **a systolic blood pressure of 140mmHg or higher or**
» **a diastolic blood pressure of 90mmHg or higher when measured on more than two occasions by a health professional using standard blood pressure-monitoring devices.**

These arbitrary thresholds used to define hypertension do not mean that if your systolic pressure is 139mmHg when you see your doctor, your blood vessels are not under stress. In fact, there is a continuous relationship between the level of tension in your arteries and the likelihood of heart attacks, strokes and kidney disease. Any reduction in blood pressure will lower the risk of complications, even if you don't have high blood pressure levels.

Because blood pressures are generally higher when you go to see your doctor, lower blood pressure thresholds are used to define hypertension using at-home monitoring or using ambulatory monitoring:

» a systolic blood pressure of 135mmHg or higher or
» a diastolic blood pressure of 85mmHg or higher.

Using these criteria, three out of four adults with type 2 diabetes will have hypertension or need medication to prevent it.

Why is hypertension so common in people with type 2 diabetes?

Regardless of how it is defined, hypertension is at least twice as common in people who have diabetes as in those who do not. Diabetes has direct effects on blood vessels to increase the tension within their walls, including:

» increased activity of the pathways that cause constriction of arteries
» increased responsiveness to these 'constrictor' signals
» reduced responsiveness to signals that cause dilation of arteries.

A number of other factors also contribute to high rates of hypertension in people with diabetes, including:

» *Ageing.* As you get older, systolic blood pressure levels gradually rise by about 1mmHg every two to three years of your adult life. By the time you retire, on average the systolic blood pressure is at least 20mmHg higher than when you were in your twenties. This is thought to be caused by progressive hardening of the arteries as the systolic blood pressure is more affected than diastolic pressure. This process is enhanced in people with diabetes and pre-diabetes. In effect this means that people with diabetes have arteries that are older than their numerical age.

» *Ethnicity.* Many of the populations at greatest risk of type 2 diabetes also have increased rates of high blood pressure. For example, people of African, Hispanic, Polynesian and other indigenous origins are at least twice as likely to develop hypertension if they also get diabetes.

» *Genes.* Blood pressure levels are influenced by your genetic make-up. High blood pressure tends to run in some families. The same families may also be prone to develop diabetes. Indeed, a family history of high blood pressure, especially at an early age, is a risk factor for type 2 diabetes and vice versa.

» *Obesity.* As discussed in Chapter 4, an enlarging waistline has a number of effects to raise the blood pressure and make it difficult to bring down. The dramatic effect of bariatric surgery on blood pressure levels stands as a testament to how important sustained weight loss is for the control of blood pressure in people with type 2 diabetes.

» *Kidney disease.* The kidneys are key regulators of blood pressure in the body because they control the amount of fluid in the system. If kidney function is impaired, as is often the case in people with type 2 diabetes (see Chapter 13) more fluid is retained and, just like too much air inside a balloon, the tension on the walls is also increased.

Reducing your blood pressure — diet and lifestyle

There are many simple things that you can do to prevent the development of high blood pressure. These are equally applicable to the many people who already have high blood pressure, in whom diet and lifestyle changes cannot only lower blood pressure levels but also reduce the need for medication(s) and improve their effectiveness. Many of these interventions are also beneficial to people with type 2 diabetes beyond their actions on blood pressure control, and are discussed in greater detail elsewhere in this book. Among the most important are:

» *Weight control (see Chapter 4).* Losing a few kilos can make a real difference to many aspects of your health, including your blood pressure. For every 1kg (2¼lb) of weight you lose, your systolic blood pressure will go down on average by approximately 1 to 2mmHg (e.g. losing 10kg/22lb in weight will usually lower your blood pressure by 10–20mmHg, which is as much as would be achieved by taking blood pressure-lowering medications). Some of this benefit to blood pressure may disappear with time, however, especially if the weight goes back on.

» *Regular physical activity.* If your blood pressure is normal, regular physical exercise can reduce the chance that it will rise as you age. In those with high blood pressure, getting regular exercise can lower your blood pressure and improve your response to blood pressure-lowering medications. There are many different forms of exercise that will work on blood pressure. The most effective programs include an element of aerobic exercise like brisk walking, climbing stairs, jogging, bicycling and swimming. Where appropriate, it is recommended that everyone with diabetes tries to get at least 30 minutes of aerobic exercise on all or most days of the week. Like the effect of weight loss, the blood pressure benefit is not sustained if you don't keep it up.

» *Smoking cessation.* Smoking is a catastrophe for people with type 2 diabetes. If the risk of heart disease, strokes and other complications was not already increased, smoking significantly kicks it along. One of the many reasons for this is that smoking raises blood pressure levels. The nicotine contained in tobacco acts to constrict blood vessels. During each cigarette, blood pressure levels rise between 20 and 30mmHg. Even though they may fall again when you are not smoking, these surges in blood pressure are extremely damaging to blood vessels and the heart.

» *A diet rich in fruit and vegetables* can also help control blood pressure. Use them to replace high fat or high calorie foods that are associated with higher blood pressure levels.

» *A diet rich in oily fish and omega-3 oils* can reduce your blood pressure. Including oily fish in your weight-loss diet can also help reduce blood pressure more effectively than weight loss or fish intake alone. Fish oil supplements can also reduce blood pressure but they need to be regularly taken in very large amounts (e.g. greater than 5g a day) to have a substantial effect. These doses are not easy to stomach because of the fishy aftertaste, and it can be hard to sustain taking this large a number of pills over a long period of time.

» *A diet rich in fibre.* Current recommendations say you should aim for at least 30g of total fibre each day. On average most people with diabetes consume less than half this amount, mostly as breakfast cereal and bread. Just by replacing refined products with wholegrain equivalents you can more than double your intake of total and soluble fibre. For those who find dietary change difficult, there are now a number of simple and highly palatable fibre supplements. Regular use of fibre supplements has been shown to have a number of useful effects in people with diabetes, including lowering blood pressure levels (see Chapter 3).

» *Stopping alcohol excesses.* Excessive alcohol intake (more than five standard drinks per day) is linked to the development of high blood pressure. For many reasons, including blood pressure, it is worth limiting your alcohol intake to no more than two standard drinks each day for men, or one standard drink each day for women (see pp. 156–157). If you can keep to these targets, then there is no reason to stop alcohol altogether. But sometimes it is easy for old habits to re-emerge, and for one glass to become another, and another ... In such circumstances it can be better to quit while you're ahead.

» *Not too much caffeine.* Caffeine is the most widely consumed stimulant in the world. Caffeine is found in coffee, tea and many 'energy' drinks, and acts by blocking receptors in the brain whose job it is to dull your brain's activity. So by preventing dulling, it stimulates the brain. This stimulation also modestly increases systolic blood pressure levels. The effect on blood pressure is most pronounced in non-coffee drinkers and immediately after having a cup. A moderate daily intake of coffee (two to three cups a day) is not associated with an increased risk of high blood pressure, mostly as you quickly become tolerant of its effects. However, a higher intake (more than five to eight cups a day or more than three espressos every day) seems to be more of an issue, especially in those who already have problems with high blood pressure.

» *Deal with daily stress.* Stress is an unavoidable part of modern life, be it physical, environmental, mental or spiritual stress. But chronic activation of stress response pathways leads to higher blood pressure, especially in those whose blood pressure is already difficult to control. Indeed, the increases in blood pressure seen in most people as they get older are not seen in those who live stress-free lives (such as cloistered nuns). This suggests that accumulated stress may be at the core of many blood pressure problems. Interventions to reduce or manage stress, such as relaxation, meditation, avoidance, disclosure and support networks, can all be very effective in some people (see Chapter 16).

Medications to lower blood pressure

Medications (also known as **anti-hypertensive agents**) are needed by over two-thirds of people with type 2 diabetes to control their blood pressure levels. There are many different types of anti-hypertensive drugs. All can be effective in lowering blood pressure. The choice of which one(s) to prescribe depends on your individual requirements.

Angiotensin-converting enzyme (ACE) inhibitors

ACE inhibitors are the most commonly used agents for blood pressure control in people with type 2 diabetes. There are many different types, brand names and manufacturers. However, what they do have in common is that the technical or generic name of ACE inhibitors usually ends in the suffix '-pril'.

ACE inhibitors came about by chance. The first ACE inhibitor was generated on the basis of chemicals found in the venom of the Amazonian pit viper, *Bothrops jararaca*, which lowered the blood pressure of its prey before devouring it.

ACE inhibitors all act to inhibit the angiotensin-converting enzyme (ACE), whose job it is to generate 'constrictor' signals in blood vessels and break down molecules that might signal blood vessels to relax. Consequently, by inhibiting ACE, blood vessels are able to dilate more easily and tension/pressure within them falls. ACE inhibitors also appear to have beneficial effects in diabetes beyond lowering blood pressure, especially in the heart, eyes and kidneys. This may be because the same signals that ACE inhibitors modify in blood vessels are also important for the development and progression of diabetic complications.

ACE inhibitors are generally well tolerated with only a few side effects experienced in some people, most notably headaches, cough or tickling sensation in the throat. Some people can put up with these without needing to stop taking this medication, but for others it can be a significant problem, meaning they have to look to other kinds of medication to lower their blood pressure. Rarely, ACE inhibitors can cause allergic reactions, including rash or more serious swelling of your face, lips, tongue or throat (known as **angioedema**). This side effect is more common in African or Caribbean patients, although it is still very uncommon.

Angiotensin-receptor blockers (ARBs)

These medications also block the effects of the angiotensin, a key constrictor signal in blood vessels. But rather than inhibiting the enzyme that generates angiotensin (which is what ACE inhibitors do), these agents impede its ability to trigger constriction of blood vessels by blocking its major receptor. Like putting a protector into a power socket to prevent a child accessing it, these agents sit in the socket to stop angiotensin plugging in. These ARBs are able to sit there for a long time, usually over a day, meaning that they have prolonged blood pressure-lowering activity and once-a-day treatment is usually all that is required.

Again, there are many different formulations, brand names and manufacturers. However, what they have in common is that the generic name of angiotensin-receptor blockers usually ends in the suffix '-sartan'.

Although they have different mechanisms of actions, recent studies suggest that ACE inhibitors and ARBs are not significantly different in terms of their actions on blood pressure and protecting the heart and other organs in diabetes. However, ARBs appear to be slightly better tolerated than ACE inhibitors and do not cause cough or angioedema.

Calcium-channel blockers

These are very effective anti-hypertensive medications that reduce blood pressure by dilating blood vessels and thereby reducing resistance to blood flow. They are second only to the ACE inhibitors in their popularity for treating high blood pressure in people with type 2 diabetes, and are often used in combination with ACE inhibitors or ARBs for the management of high blood pressure. Calcium-channel blockers are especially effective in people with hardening of their arteries, where stiffness in the blood vessels drives up the systolic blood pressure.

Calcium-channel blockers are also long acting, meaning that many can provide good blood pressure control with a single daily dose. Calcium-channel blockers are generally well tolerated by people with diabetes. However, some people find swelling of the ankles, headaches, flushing and constipation troubling, especially at higher doses.

Again, there are many different formulations and manufacturers. The most common class are the dihydropyridine calcium-channel blockers, which are denoted by a generic name that ends in the suffix '-dipine'.

Diuretics

Diuretics are safe, effective and inexpensive medications that have been used for many years and have been proven to reduce blood pressure and improve health outcomes. They are more effective in combination with other anti-hypertensive agents, and are generally used this way in people with type 2 diabetes.

Diuretics make you lose more salt (and water) in your urine, thus lowering your blood pressure in the same way as releasing air from a balloon lowers its pressure. For this reason they are widely known as **water pills** or **water tablets**. Many also have modest vasodilator effects similar to the calcium-channel blockers detailed above, which may be their major mechanism of actions when given in low doses.

The low doses used by most people with diabetes mean that they seldom make you go to the toilet too frequently and/or dry you out excessively. However, higher doses of diuretics can have these drawbacks. But in most people with diabetes, especially those who also have heart failure or swollen ankles, this drying out action can also be quite beneficial and help to relieve symptoms as well as improve blood pressure control. Excessive urination can also lead to the loss of important chemicals in the urine, such as potassium and magnesium, and increase levels of uric acid which may cause gout. In some individuals, diuretics can also interfere with their glucose control.

Beta-blockers

Beta-blockers lower the blood pressure by blocking stimulation signals from the sympathetic nervous system. As detailed above, when you are nervous or stressed, activation of the sympathetic nervous system makes your heart race and beat more strongly, while the resistance vessels constrict. Being overweight or having kidney or heart disease can also activate the sympathetic nervous system and cause high blood pressure through overactivity of the same pathways. Beta-blockers prevent these signals so are able to slow the pulse, making your heart beat less forcefully. These actions are also useful not only to lower the blood pressure, but to reduce stress on the heart. Consequently beta-blockers are generally used in someone with diabetes who has angina, heart failure and some disturbances in their heart's rhythm.

As medication used to reduce the risk of heart attacks and strokes, beta-blockers are considered to be less effective overall than calcium-channel blockers, ACE inhibitors, ARBs or diuretics. Moreover, their side effect profile is not as favourable. For example, some people experience tiredness, low mood/depression, sleep disturbance, weight gain or impotence with beta-blockers. Breathing problems can also be exacerbated in some people. Beta-blockers can also interfere with glucose control and the body's response to hypoglycaemia.

However, there are some circumstances when beta-blockers are advantageous, such as in people with heart disease. They can also be used to treat glaucoma and resting tremors (e.g. troublesome shaking hands). In addition, some studies suggest that those people who are prone to sympathetic induced surges, such as after smoking, may be better protected by beta-blockers. However, such individuals would be best protected by stopping smoking.

Again, there are many different formulations and manu-facturers. However, in common, the generic name of beta-blockers usually ends in the suffix '-olol'.

All together now

Most people with type 2 diabetes will need some medication to keep their blood pressure under control. A small number will get away with just one tablet, but for the majority two or three different classes of medication will be required in combination with diet and lifestyle interventions. This is certainly worth the effort. For every 1mmHg decrease in your systolic blood pressure, the long-term risk of heart attack or stroke will fall by 2 to 3 per cent. This means that if you have high blood pressure and you can safely reduce your systolic blood pressure by 10mmHg, your risk of a heart attack or stroke will fall by 20 to 30 per cent. In fact, that sustained control of blood pressure is the most important way to protect the heart, brain and other organs in people with type 2 diabetes.

But this must be sustained. There are no 'bonus points' for once having had your blood pressure under control. For example, evidence from clinical studies in which good blood pressure control was achieved for a period of time but then lost, suggests your risk of complications from diabetes is only as good as your current blood pressure level. If you lose control, then the chance of having a heart attack or stroke will also rise. Equally, if you have had troublesome blood pressure levels and you and your doctor can find the right combination of medications and other interventions to get it under control, then the legacy of a period of poor blood pressure control can be erased.

9

Eschew the fat

UNDERSTAND

» One of the most efficient ways to reduce your risk of complications is to aim to improve the levels of fats and cholesterol in your blood (known collectively as 'lipids').

» The most widely used class of medication in the treatment of type 2 diabetes is the statins, which inhibit the manufacture of cholesterol by the liver, so LDL cholesterol levels fall in the blood by between 20 to 50 per cent.

» LDL cholesterol levels in your blood are only partly determined by the fats in your diet. The majority of the cholesterol in your bloodstream is made inside your body.

» HDL cholesterol works to remove cholesterol from your blood vessels and so protects them from atherosclerosis.

» Although diabetes can affect the level of LDL and HDL cholesterol in the blood, by far the greatest change is the overproduction of triglyceride-rich particles.

MANAGE

» Get the best out of your statin by taking it in the evening.

» Reduce the amount of saturated fat and increase the amount of soluble fibre in your diet to improve your lipid levels beyond what can be achieved by medicines alone.

» Avoid any food that contains trans fat. For people with type 2 diabetes there is no safe intake of trans fats.

» Get up and get active. This will improve many aspects of your health, including your lipid levels.

Fats are one of the most important building blocks of life. However, they can also be the foundation of poor health, especially in people with type 2 diabetes. Fat has a number of characteristics that make it unhealthy in excess. It has twice the calories of sugar or protein, so that for the same weight of fat, more goes to your waistline. Likewise, cholesterol can be a means to a sticky end by clogging the walls of blood vessels, contributing to their narrowing and stiffening, and ultimately increasing the risk of heart attacks and strokes (see chapters 10 and 15). High levels of fats and cholesterol in the blood are also associated with kidney, foot and eye disease in people with type 2 diabetes.

One of the most efficient ways to reduce your risk of complications is to aim to improve the levels of fats and cholesterol in your blood (known collectively as your **lipids**). All people with type 2 diabetes should have a blood test to look at their complete lipid profile when they are diagnosed and at regular intervals thereafter (at least annually). This blood test is

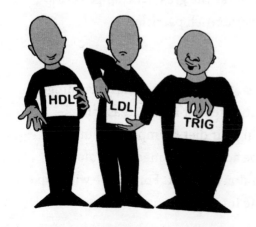

Lipids come in different sizes and densities. They are generally grouped into three main types: good, bad and ugly.

usually taken after a period of fasting (no food or drink, except water, for 12 hours), which in practical terms means first thing in the morning before any breakfast. This is so that your lipid levels aren't confused with those of your last meal. The results of this important test will be used to determine the best strategy to get your lipids under control.

Lipids are mostly transported around the body in special waterproof containers known as **lipoprotein particles** (because they are particles made up of lipids and proteins). They must be contained because oil does not dissolve in water. If you tried it, it would just congeal on the surface, where it would be unusable. The same goes for lipids. These particles come in different sizes and densities and have different functions in the body. For the purpose of your blood test, these lipid particles can be broadly classified into three basic types:

1. low density lipoproteins (LDL)
2. high density lipoproteins (HDL)
3. triglyceride-rich lipoproteins.

Why is LDL cholesterol important?

Most of the cholesterol that circulates in the bloodstream is contained in low density lipoproteins (LDL) and is therefore known as **LDL cholesterol**. The cholesterol contained in these LDL particles in generally considered to be 'bad cholesterol'. This is because high levels of LDL cholesterol are associated with an increased risk of heart attacks, strokes and other diseases of the blood vessels.

At the same time, there is good evidence that lowering LDL cholesterol can reduce this risk. For every 1mmol/L (39mg/dL) you lower your LDL cholesterol, the risk of a heart attack lowers by between 20 and 25 per cent. This is readily achievable through diet, exercise and other lifestyle changes and, for those who are at high risk, regularly taking LDL-lowering medications.

All people with type 2 diabetes should make lowering their LDL level an important priority, even if their levels are relatively normal. This is because lowering the LDL cholesterol in the blood also means lowering the amount of cholesterol in your blood vessels, and this in turn means a lower risk of heart attacks and strokes (see chapters 10 and 15).

LDL levels aren't usually any higher in people with type 2 diabetes when compared with those who don't have diabetes. However, there is often an excess of **small, dense LDL** particles. These are the 'baddest of the bad (cholesterol)' because of their increased ability to deposit cholesterol into your blood vessels and not respond to signals to return any excess cholesterol to the liver. Consequently, people with type 2 diabetes will benefit from lowering their LDL cholesterol level even if it is not too high, because it will also help eliminate these 'very bad' LDL particles.

The main job of LDL cholesterol is to transport cholesterol out of the liver and to any areas of the body that need it to build. Areas that are damaged or inflamed need more cholesterol to rebuild, so they capture LDL particles and utilise their store of cholesterol. For example, when blood vessels are stressed, damaged or inflamed they also accumulate cholesterol which they take from LDL particles. The accumulation of cholesterol in the walls of blood vessels progressively leads to narrowing and instability of blood vessels and leads to heart attacks and strokes.

Too much bad (or very bad) cholesterol in your blood means that cholesterol can be taken up into your blood vessels more easily and in greater amounts. But if you can successfully lower your LDL cholesterol, it means that the important triggers to accumulate cholesterol in the blood vessels, like diabetes or high blood pressure, have much less to work with. And this means less heart disease.

How can you lower LDL cholesterol?

The great majority of the cholesterol in your bloodstream is made inside your body. Cholesterol is an important component of healthy function, so the human body has enzymes to make the cholesterol it thinks it needs. Each day, you usually make about 1000mg of cholesterol, and take in another 250mg from your diet. The body even recycles cholesterol from the bile in your intestines so there is no unnecessary wastage.

This means that LDL cholesterol levels in your blood are only partly determined by what you eat. But it also means that blood levels can rise to dangerous levels if your liver makes too much LDL cholesterol, even if fatty foods never touch your lips. Consequently, reducing your LDL cholesterol is all about reducing the amount of cholesterol made by the liver, while at the same time improving your diet.

There are many different **lipid-lowering medications** that act to reduce the amount of cholesterol made by the body and reduce LDL cholesterol levels in the blood.

Most people with type 2 diabetes will need lipid-lowering medications to keep their LDL cholesterol levels as low as possible.

The most widely used type of medication to treat lipids is the **statins**. Statins work by partly inhibiting the manufacture of cholesterol by the liver. To make up for the shortfall, the liver then actively takes back any harmful cholesterol from the bloodstream and tissues. So LDL cholesterol levels fall in the blood by between 20 and 50 per cent.

There are many different brands and formulations of various products, and these are often different in different countries. Each has a chemical (generic) name that ends with the sufffix '-statin'. A number of different statins are currently available, including:

» atorvastatin
» fluvastatin
» lovastatin
» pitavastatin
» pravastatin
» rosuvastatin
» simvastatin.

These chemical names are usually displayed on the packet under the brand name in smaller writing. Each of these statins will reduce LDL levels, although they vary in how much it will be reduced and their side effects (see below).

Statins were first identified by Japanese biochemists looking at chemicals made by fungi to defend themselves against other organisms. They discovered that some of these chemicals also blocked the ability to make cholesterol, and these became the first statins. Other fungi, including oyster mushrooms and red yeast *koji* (a traditional Chinese dish in which rice is fermented in the presence of a specific red mould), also naturally contain a statin, and consequently have the ability to modestly lower cholesterol levels in the blood.

Some people cannot take statins because of troublesome side effects. The most common problems are muscle aches and pains, which are experienced by over one-third of people taking statins, especially those people on high doses. The risk of muscle pain is partly genetically determined because some people do not have the ability to break down statins efficiently. There is no easy means to prevent muscle aches and pains with a statin. The response is not the same for all statins, meaning that if you have muscle pains with one statin it does not mean you will have the same problems with another statin. So your doctor will often ask you to try another statin if the side effects from one are troublesome. However, many people either have to use smaller doses of a statin, where symptoms are better tolerated, or discontinue it altogether. Recent studies suggest statins may modestly increase the risk of diabetes. However, statins themselves have no major effects on the glucose control of people who already have diabetes.

There are a number of ways to get the best effect out of your statin and maximise your reduction of LDL cholesterol.

Good timing

Statins are usually taken once a day. However, most cholesterol production by the liver occurs at night. So the most efficient way to reduce cholesterol production is to take your statin in the evening. This can add a further 10 per cent reduction to LDL cholesterol levels. The other advantage of taking your statin at night is that the peak chemical concentration coincides with the time you are least likely to experience side effects, when you are asleep.

Ezetimibe

While statins tell the liver to make less cholesterol, the body tries to make up the shortfall by extracting more cholesterol from your intestines (both that contained in your food and the bile released to digest it). So LDL cholesterol levels don't fall by as much as they could. Taking ezetimibe tablets effectively halves the reabsorption of cholesterol. It doesn't do much on its own, but in those already taking a statin, taking ezetimibe as well can reduce LDL cholesterol levels by a further 20 to 25 per cent. Some statins now come mixed with ezetimibe in the same capsule, so that using ezetimibe may not mean taking any extra pills.

Sterols

Some foods contain natural chemicals with a structure very similar to cholesterol (known as **plant sterols/stanols** or **phytosterols/stanols**). This means they are able to compete with cholesterol for absorption from the intestine, so that less cholesterol is taken up from your diet. Sterols are naturally high in many vegetable oils, nuts and legumes, which can be effectively used as a meat substitute in an everyday diet. But sufficient naturally occurring sterols are hard to get while at the same time trying to limit your overall food intake. So a number of companies have deliberately enriched their foods with sterols to increase their potential health benefits, including margarines, yoghurts, salad dressings, cheeses, breads and even orange juice. These can be hard to find in the shops and tend to be more expensive than standard products, but will further lower your LDL cholesterol levels. Plant sterol supplements are also available from health food stores. Both supplements and fortified foods only have a modest effect and work best when taken regularly in combination with statins and in high doses (more than 2g per day).

Dietary fibre

A diet high in fibre, and in particular **soluble fibre**, can also have beneficial effects on LDL cholesterol levels, as well as a number of other health issues. It is thought that soluble fibre causes the liver to make more bile acids from cholesterol, thereby diverting it away from making LDL cholesterol. Dietary fibre can be obtained from a variety of sources, especially wholegrain cereals, fruit and vegetables as well as from nutritional supplements (see Chapter 3).

A low cholesterol diet

Most people can only lower their LDL cholesterol by 5 to 10 per cent at best when going 'cholesterol-free' in their diet. However, in people who are already taking lipid-lowering medications, the machinery to capture cholesterol from the intestine is significantly ramped up. It is recommended that all those on a statin should also limit their intake of cholesterol-rich foods, including:

» Meat and dairy. Any meat that contains high levels of animal fat will also contain cholesterol, especially those parts that are visibly fatty, such as the skin and the liver. Substituting lean cuts or vegetable protein (like legumes) is one useful way to lower your LDL cholesterol levels.

» Some low fat foods are paradoxically high in cholesterol, including egg yolks, coconut, palm oils and prawns/shrimp. Reducing your intake of these can also lower your LDL cholesterol levels.

» Most foods will now have a label stating how much cholesterol the food contains. Read the label and where possible pick the product that contains the lowest amount of cholesterol.

A low fat diet

LDL cholesterol levels are also partly determined by the mix of fats in your diet. Fats come in many forms. Most have three chains of fatty acids lined up like cricket stumps and linked at the top by glycerol, like the bails. If you don't play cricket, you could say it looks like the letter 'E'. This complex is called a **triglyceride** (because of its three — tri — chains). Over 90 per cent of the fats you eat, and almost all that you store in the body, are in the form of triglycerides. The length of the stumps (fatty acid chains) and the type of bonds between adjacent carbons determine its physical properties and its role in the body.

If a fat contains the maximum possible number of hydrogen atoms, it is said to be (fully) **saturated**. This chemical arrangement results in a straightening of its molecular structure, allowing it to pack in tightly. This means it can be solid on the knife, but easily melts with a small amount of heat on your toast. It also means saturated fats have a greater energy density than unsaturated fat. For this reason, most of the fat you store in the body is in the form of saturated fat, which is slowly broken down between meals to ensure a constant energy supply.

Unsaturated fats are those that have (one or many) double bonds, which effectively introduces a kink into their structure that prevents them from stacking efficiently. This makes them more difficult to make solid, so they are generally liquid (an oil) at room temperature. But in your body, unsaturated fats also mean more flexibility.

Most foods contain a mixture of saturated and unsaturated fats. Foods that are rich in saturated fat are also often high in cholesterol. But in addition, eating saturated fat also triggers an increase in LDL cholesterol levels in the blood.

So any foods that are high in saturated fat will be able to increase your cholesterol levels even if they claim to be 'cholesterol-free'.

Equally, LDL cholesterol can be lowered by reducing your intake of foods that are high in saturated fats, including:

» Limit full-fat dairy products (especially whole milk, yoghurt, cheese and ice-cream) and/or substituting low fat varieties instead.

» Choose lean cuts of meat and remove all visible fat before cooking. The meat of grass-fed animals and free-range birds also contains lower levels of saturated fat than the conventional bulk (grain) fed stocks.

» Eat skinless chicken.

» Where practical, substitute animal protein with vegetable protein, e.g. substitute legumes for mince so you use half as much mince in your spaghetti bolognese.

» Substitute animal meats with seafood and fish.

» Limit your intake of eggs, especially egg yolks. Up to five eggs a week may be acceptable for people with diabetes as part of a healthy diet. But for those with high LDL levels, further moderation should be considered.

» Limit your intake of processed foods, which often contain a significant amount of hidden fat with the addition of butter, oils and lower quality non-lean meat (e.g. pies, pasties, fish and chips, commercial cakes and biscuits/cookies).

» Limit your use of butter in cooking and/or use margarine rich in polyunsaturated or monounsaturated fat.

» Where possible, cook without oil. Where oils are necessary, use products rich in **monounsaturated fats** (MUFAs) such as those found in Mediterranean countries. These are also associated with lower LDL cholesterol levels. Whether this is a direct effect or just because MUFAs replace saturated fat in the diet is still unclear. The most common MUFA in the Mediterranean diet is **oleic acid**, which is found in vegetable and seed oils, nuts, avocado and some meats. Tea oil and olive oil contain more MUFAs than normal canola oils, which are in turn greater than sunflower, peanut, corn and soybean oils. However, on the market now are many oil products which are naturally high in oleic acid (greater than

70g per 100g, or 70 per cent) and comparable in content to olive oils.

Avoid trans fats

Trans fats are an unnatural form of unsaturated fat that has been realigned with a straight backbone. This means that even though it is unsaturated, it looks and behaves more like the straight chain of a saturated fat. Most trans fats are deliberately created during the processing of vegetable oils (by hydrogenation) to make them solid at room temperature, melt on baking (or eating) and more resistant to going off (rancid) when compared to animal fats like butter. Prolonged deep-frying can also generate trans fats, which are then transferred to the foods you are eating.

Trans fats increase heart disease partly by raising bad (LDL) cholesterol levels and lowering good (HDL) cholesterol levels and increasing levels of inflammation. Saturated fat does the same thing, but trans fats are much more potent. In fact, for the same amount, trans fats increase the risk of heart disease more than any other component of your diet. This is not just the case for those who eat a lot of them — even a small intake may be sufficient to begin increasing your risk of heart disease. There appears to be no safe limit for trans fats. However, in many Western societies 2 to 3 per cent of all calories are now delivered as trans fats.

The only real way to avoid trans fats is to avoid foods containing them, or choose foods in which the processing has specifically prevented their formation. Major sources of trans fats are deep-fried fast foods, bakery products, packaged snack foods, fried foods and baked goods. Steer clear of any processed foods that have any trans fats listed on their nutritional contents.

What is good cholesterol and how can you get more?

Not all cholesterol is bad. About 20 to 30 per cent of cholesterol in the blood is contained in small, dense packages known as high-density lipoproteins (HDL). HDL particles perform a number of jobs that are important for the health of blood vessels, including:

» soaking up excess cholesterol from the walls of blood vessels and transporting it back to the liver for excretion, storage or recycling (known as **reverse cholesterol transport**)

» transferring their signalling proteins to other particles, which allows them to dump their fatty cargo safely back into the liver, rather than getting stuck in your blood vessels

» HDL also contains antioxidant molecules and may also have beneficial effects on clotting and inflammation.

These helpful actions partly explain why **HDL cholesterol** is considered to be **'good cholesterol'**. Certainly, people with high levels of HDL cholesterol have a lower risk of heart disease and strokes, and those with low HDL levels have more problems with cholesterol deposits in their blood vessels.

HDL cholesterol levels are often low in people with type 2 diabetes. This is partly because HDL particles get used up faster when trying to deal with all the other changes in fat metabolism.

Many of the things you are already doing as part of your routine diabetes management will be improving your HDL cholesterol levels, as well of other aspects of your health. These include:

» *Losing excess waist.* Being overweight or obese is associated with reduced HDL cholesterol levels. Every 1kg (2¼lb) in weight you can lose means a better waistline and better cholesterol (see Chapter 4).

» *Increasing your level of physical activity* will increase HDL levels, especially in those with low levels. Regular aerobic exercise seems to have the best effect. This action seems to correlate with the ability of exercise to help you lose weight. However, it is not instantaneous and it may take many months to see any significant change in HDL. But then, good things take time.

» *Stopping smoking* is important for many reasons, one of which is its impact on HDL cholesterol. Smokers have lower HDL levels, while stopping smoking will increase HDL levels by 10 to 20 per cent on average.

» *Drinking alcohol, in moderation.* It is well known that those who regularly drink a modest amount of alcohol have slightly higher HDL cholesterol levels when compared to those who don't drink at all or drink only occasionally. This may partly explain why the risk of heart attacks and strokes is also a little lower in drinkers when compared to teetotallers. No one particular type of beverage (beer, wine or spirits) appears to provide more benefit than another, but there may be some extra benefit in consuming alcohol with meals. The best HDL levels and the best health are seen in those who have a regular intake of 5 to 10g of alcohol each day. In some countries, any drinks that contain alcohol have on their label how much alcohol they contain; this is often expressed as the number of 'standard drinks', and one standard drink is equivalent to 10g of alcohol. So a bottle of wine will contain around eight standard drinks. Of course, the amount you might drink in each glass may be much more than one standard drink, and this should be taken into account when working out the safe drinking amount for yourself.

It is generally recommended that all men should drink no more than 40g of alcohol per day; women are recommended to drink no more than half this amount (i.e. 20g of alcohol per day) to gain the benefits of alcohol without its health risks. But this does not mean that non-drinkers should start drinking alcohol to raise their HDL, especially now they have diabetes. A little tipple can easily become more if the bottle is just there. It is far healthier to never drink at all than go down this slippery slope. Irregular heavy drinking bouts, even if accompanied by usual moderation, can undo any benefits and contribute to high blood pressure and hypoglycaemia in some people on glucose-lowering medications. Alcohol is also a good source of excess calories (just think 'beer belly').

» *Substituting unsaturated fats* into your diet (instead of eating saturated and trans fats) will also help raise your HDL cholesterol levels.

Because of the importance of HDL, a number of different medicines have been developed to try to raise HDL cholesterol, especially in those with type 2 diabetes. These include niacin (vitamin B3) and fibrates. At the present time, though, there is no evidence that their specific actions on HDL cholesterol confer any significant benefits in people with diabetes. Moreover, niacin can raise glucose levels in some people with diabetes. Other potentially useful actions of these agents on triglycerides are discussed below.

What are triglycerides doing in your blood?

The most important store of energy in the human body is fat. As discussed in Chapter 2, this energy store is mostly in the form of triglycerides, which you bank in your fatty tissues under your skin and around your waistline. When you are eating, these energy stores are built up. But when you are not eating these stores are slowly broken down and used to provide the energy for life.

Because fat doesn't dissolve in water, to reach our stores it must be transported in large triglyceride-rich particles. Most triglycerides are made by the liver, which converts any excess energy in the diet into triglycerides, packages it into particles and ships it off into the bloodstream so it can be dumped into our fat stores. These particles are made up of mostly triglycerides, with some cholesterol and very little protein, so they have a very low density (and are therefore also called very low density particles or **VLDL cholesterol**). Excess fat in your diet also needs to be packaged and sent off. After digestion, the intestine packages fat for the body in a different kind of very, very low density particle (known as a **chylomicron**).

Although type 2 diabetes can affect the level of LDL and HDL cholesterol in your blood, by far the greatest change in your lipid levels is the over-production of these ugly triglyceride-rich particles. This is because insulin does much more than just look after your glucose levels.

After a meal, when there is lots of glucose, this is the time to build up your fuel stores. So insulin also signals the body to take up triglycerides as well as glucose, and store them until their energy is needed later. Insulin also signals the liver to stop making new triglyceride-rich particles. After all, you have just eaten. In the same way, and for the same reasons, it also tells it to stop making glucose.

When insulin levels are low, such as between meals, triglycerides are broken down and released into the bloodstream. This is important for two main reasons. First, triglycerides are used by the liver to make new glucose and thus sustain blood glucose levels for the sake of your brain. Second, this fat provides an alternate fuel source for the working of your muscles, liver, heart and many other organs. Many others that is, except for your brain, which cannot use fat so gets preferential treatment. When other organs use fat for their metabolism, this frees up glucose for your brain.

However, in those with diabetes there is not enough insulin (function) to keep metabolism under control. So not only do glucose levels rise, but there is also not enough insulin to support the healthy uptake of fat or to stop the liver, which keeps cranking out triglyceride-rich particles. This means that triglyceride levels are elevated in the blood of people with type 2 diabetes as well as glucose, especially after meals. People with diabetes are two to three times more likely to have elevated blood triglycerides (more than 2mmol/L or 177mg/dL) than people without diabetes. These triglyceride-rich particles are bad for you in a number of ways:

»   HDL particles get used up trying to deal with them, so as triglyceride levels rise, levels of good (HDL) cholesterol fall.

»   Because of their large size, these triglyceride-rich particles are prone to get stuck in the walls of blood vessels, which contributes to atherosclerosis and ultimately heart attacks and strokes (see chapters 10 and 15).

»   In extreme cases, these lipid particles are deposited under the skin as itchy, whitish lumps, known as xanthomas.

How can you lower your triglyceride levels?

Again, many of the things you are already doing as part of your routine diabetes management will be improving your triglyceride levels, as well as other aspects of your health. These include:

» losing excess weight
» regular physical activity
» achieving and maintaining good glucose control
» reducing the saturated fat in your diet
» avoiding trans fats in your diet.

In addition, there may be other things you can do to keep your triglycerides down that you might not immediately think of doing, including the following.

Avoiding sweetened beverages

Fructose is present in many carbonated beverages and fruit juice mixes, and it is added to many prepared foods as a preservative and sweetener. Immediately following the intake of high-fructose drinks, triglyceride levels can rise quite dramatically. In those with already elevated levels and/or difficulty clearing away triglycerides, these sweet drinks can still be a cause of rising lipid levels, even when they contain no fat.

Increased intake of omega-3 fatty acids

Fats are more than just the means to a sticky end. Some fats are also essential for good health, and must be found in the diet. The most well known of these are the **omega-3** polyunsaturated fatty acids, of which the most important nutritionally are alpha-linolenic acid (ALA) from plants, and eicosapentaenoic acid (EPA) and docosahexaenoic acid (DHA), which are found in high levels in oily fish. It is recommended that people with diabetes consume a meal of oily fish (such as salmon, herring, mackerel, anchovies, sardines and to a lesser extent tuna) two or three times every week, to keep up their omega-3s. Although enjoyable for some, many find that this is difficult to achieve. These doses generally will not be enough to lower triglycerides, although they can have other beneficial effects. If you can't get enough from fish, eating fortified foods with added amounts of omega-3 fat can prove useful, including bread, mayonnaise, yoghurt, orange juice, pasta, milk, eggs, infant formula and even ice-cream.

Many people also take supplements that contain the required amounts of omega-3, such as **fish oils** and **flaxseed (linseed) oil**. Clinical trials have demonstrated that fish oil supplements can lower blood triglyceride levels in people with diabetes by about one-third. However, the dose required to achieve any significant change in your triglyceride levels is high (more than 2g per day) and can leave a 'fishy' aftertaste. But while triglycerides are strongly associated with all the complications of diabetes, it also remains to be established whether omega-3 supplements actually reduce your chances of developing these complications.

Moderation of alcohol

Those people who regularly drink heavily often have elevated triglyceride levels. This partly reflects the extra calories that come with drinking as well as the direct effects of alcohol. Some of this rise in triglycerides will improve once any excessive alcohol intake is stopped.

Because of the potentially toxic effects of triglyceride-rich particles, the potential value of medications to target this kind of lipid have been widely studied in people with type 2 diabetes. The best studied are the **fibrates**. Again, there are many different brands and formulations of different products, and these often vary in different countries. Each has a chemical (generic) name that contains the letters 'fibr'. Only three fibrates are currently available, including:

» fenofibrate

» gemfibrozil

» bezafibrate.

These are able to lower triglyceride levels by 20 to 40 per cent in people with type 2 diabetes, when used on top of standard treatment with a statin and other dietary modifications detailed above. In people with high triglyceride levels, treatment with a fibrate has been shown to prevent heart attacks. It also may reduce the risk of eye, nerve and foot complications. Fenofibrate can be used in people who are taking a statin, so is the preferred fibrate for people with type 2 diabetes. Gemfibrozil may interact with your statin in a way to increase the risk of side effects including muscle pain and damage, so is only used on its own, in people who can't use a statin.

10

Diabetes in my heart

UNDERSTAND

» Heart attacks are a common complication of type 2 diabetes, and are sadly the major cause of death.

» Good management of your diabetes is able to reduce your chance of having a heart attack by over half.

» Heart attacks are caused by the erosion of an unstable surface of a blood vessel supplying the heart, which causes it to become completely blocked by a clot.

» Many heart attacks in people with type 2 diabetes are silent. The first sign may be shortness of breath, ankle swelling or other signs of heart failure.

» The changes in your blood vessels that lead to a heart attack are reversible when the risk factors for atherosclerosis are addressed.

MANAGE

» Get your levels of bad (LDL) cholesterol as low as possible. Even if your levels are not high, less cholesterol means less chance of heart disease.

» Treat high blood pressure levels and maintain smooth control over them.

» Stop smoking as a matter of priority and encourage others

in your environment to do the same as it may also affect your health.

» Undertake a comprehensive risk factor assessment with the help of your diabetes care team to calculate your individual risk of a heart attack, and the benefits that can be achieved from each treatment.

» Become familiar with the warning signs of a heart attack. Have an action plan for what to do in the event of a heart attack and when to call for an ambulance.

All parts of the body depend on the flow of blood for their survival. If this flow is blocked, even for a brief period, any parts downstream from the blockage suffer and may die. When this blockage occurs in the blood vessels that supply the heart (known as the **coronary arteries**) it is called a **heart attack** (also known as **myocardial infarction** or **MI**). When a blockage occurs in blood flow to the brain it is called a **stroke** (also known as a **cerebrovascular accident**; see Chapter 15). Together, heart attacks and strokes may be the most important complications of having type 2 diabetes, accounting for over two-thirds of all deaths in people with diabetes.

The burden of heart disease among patients with type 2 diabetes is substantial. Many years of life are lost, while quality of life for survivors is greatly reduced. Between one-third to half of all adults with type 2 diabetes will have heart disease. Approximately 1 to 3 per cent of people with type 2 diabetes experience heart attacks and strokes every year. Overall, this risk is at least twice that observed in people who do not have diabetes.

Finding ways to prevent or reverse this process is therefore an integral part of diabetes care.

And it does work! If you have diabetes today, the risk of having a heart attack or stroke is less than half what it was for those with type 2 diabetes twenty years ago. With modern diabetes care, it is anticipated that heart attack rates will continue to fall. This chapter will look at the key opportunities you have to look after your heart and, with it, your life.

What causes heart attacks?

Think of your blood vessels as roads that allow for the steady flow of traffic along major arterials to smaller streets and then back again in a round trip. Like any carriageway, the health of these roads is important for maintaining this flow. If the surface stays flat, traffic flows smoothly and easily gets to where it needs to go. However, over long periods of time, changes are occurring under the surface of our roads, causing them to thicken and soften. This is known as **atherosclerosis** and is the start of the process that eventually leads to heart attacks and strokes.

These changes do not occur equally in all parts of the road. Streets that get damaged fastest are the ones that have the extra pressure of heavy trucks or turning vehicles. The same occurs in our arteries, where the large blood vessels under the greatest pressure are most vulnerable, especially where vessels divide and blood flow turns a corner into the heart or the brain. When atherosclerosis affects the coronary blood vessels that supply the heart, it is known as **coronary heart disease** or **CHD**.

Years may go by as the structures underneath the surface become progressively unstable in spots. The surface may even start to bulge a little bit (known as **plaque**). But still the surface remains intact and the traffic keeps flowing. Then one fateful day, usually after a particularly large truck passes (or another stressful event), the surface breaks and a pothole occurs. The next car falls into the pothole. The car behind it hits the first car and a major pile-up ensues, completely blocking the road. This is precisely what happens if you have a heart attack. A coronary artery becomes clotted because of an erosion or rupture of its protective surface.

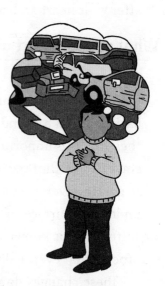

Think of your blood vessels as roads that allow for the steady flow of traffic. A heart attack is a major pile-up that blocks the road to your heart.

In most people with diabetes, a heart attack or stroke is the first sign that there is anything wrong with their arteries.

If this blockage can't be quickly cleared, then everything further down the road relying on the traffic getting through will suffer. Unlike damage to your skin, heart muscle and brain cells cannot grow back, so any significant loss of blood flow always means some permanent loss of function. But if the clot is dissolved and traffic flow can be quickly restored, any permanent damage can be prevented or kept to a minimum.

Sometimes surface erosions and ruptures are limited and the resulting clot is so small that any obstruction is partial. Such events do not cause a heart attack, as sufficient blood flow is still maintained along the artery for the heart to survive. But as each clot is incorporated into the wall, the road is progressively narrowed and further compromised in its ability to handle more than a trickle of traffic.

Of course with a road, if you lose a lane or two things only really come to a head at 'rush hour', when more traffic wants to use the road. The same occurs when the heart needs more blood flow, such as with physical exertion or other stresses that get the heart racing. In such circumstances any narrowing in the coronary artery can suddenly become limiting. This is experienced as chest pain (known as **angina**) and is often a forerunner of more complete and more serious blockages in the future.

What is your risk of a heart attack?

Although having diabetes increases your risk of heart attacks, the personal risk for a heart attack varies considerably between people with diabetes. In younger people with diabetes, their risk is quite small, so even with the doubling in risk associated with having diabetes this doesn't add up to much. However, for older individuals with type 2 diabetes, or those with other risk factors such as high blood pressure, high total cholesterol or smokers, any doubling in their (already elevated) risk caused by diabetes has a much more substantial effect in absolute terms.

It is recommended that all people with type 2 diabetes should undergo comprehensive risk factor assessment with the help of their diabetes care team to identify whether more intensive management can result in the greatest absolute benefits. A range of different 'risk calculators' is available. Each combines a number of key factors to estimate your personal risk of having a heart attack. Your doctor will be able to plug into these various factors about your history, your symptoms and signs, as well as results of your blood tests to calculate your personal risk.

While these calculators can be used to inform you about your risks, more importantly they can be used to estimate the benefits that could be achieved from interventions designed to lower your risk (see below). For example, if prescribing lipid-lowering medication to reduce your cholesterol levels is able to reduce your risk of having a heart attack by 20 to 25 per cent, then the risk in someone who has a 5 per cent risk of a heart attack in the next 5 years is reduced by this medication to around 4 per cent. In absolute terms the 1 per cent reduction is quite small and may not be worth the side effects or the cost of the medication. By comparison, for someone who has a 50 per cent risk of a heart attack, lipid-lowering medication has over ten times the benefit (by reducing their risk by over 10 per cent in absolute terms, to less than 40 per cent). In this situation, more aggressive treatment and targets have greater gains — more bang for your buck. In this way it is possible to put real numbers on what you are achieving with management of your diabetes.

How to prevent heart attacks

The scenario of progressive change under the surface of your blood vessels, eventually leading to their loss of integrity, is preventable. In fact, it may even be partly reversible. There are now a number of different opportunities to look after your blood vessels and keep their traffic flowing for many years to come. Some of these opportunities include:

Reducing the LDL cholesterol levels in the blood

Large deposits of cholesterol under the surface of our blood vessels are the most important reason why blood vessels become weak and eventually break down. A number of different factors cause cholesterol to accumulate in the walls of the coronary arteries. Most of this cholesterol comes from the LDL cholesterol present in the blood (see Chapter 9). This is also known as the 'bad cholesterol' because of its strong association with heart disease. Even though most people with type 2 diabetes do not have very elevated LDL cholesterol levels, by reducing your circulating levels of LDL cholesterol you also reduce the risk of a heart attack or stroke. For every 1mmol/L (39mg/dL) you lower your LDL cholesterol, your risk will fall by 20 to 25 per cent. This can be readily achieved with a combination of diet, physical activity and appropriate use of lipid-lowering medications.

Raising the HDL cholesterol in the blood

The body has a way to safely transport cholesterol out of blood vessels and back into the liver. This is performed by HDL cholesterol particles (also known as 'good cholesterol'), which is discussed in detail in Chapter 9. Diabetes reduces HDL levels, meaning that this beneficial action is also reduced in people with diabetes. The higher your HDL cholesterol the greater your capacity to offset the effects of bad cholesterol, particularly with regards to the development and progression of heart disease, so that individuals with the highest levels of HDL cholesterol have a lower risk of heart disease and strokes. There are a number of different ways to increase HDL levels, mainly through a combination of a healthy diet, physical activity and appropriate use of lipid-lowering medication.

Reducing elevated triglycerides in the blood

The greatest change in lipid levels in the blood associated with diabetes is the increase in triglycerides. In those with elevated triglyceride levels (greater than 2mmol/L or 177mg/dL), treatment with the triglyceride-lowering drug fenofibrate is able to reduce the risk of heart attacks. It does not appear to have the same benefits in people who do not have high triglycerides or in those who already have heart disease. However, it may have other beneficial effects for your eyes and your feet.

Reducing systolic blood pressure

The tension on the walls of our arteries is just like the pressure of traffic on the surface of a road: the greater and heavier the traffic, the more likely that the road will become progressively damaged and potholes will eventually occur. One simple way to keep our blood vessels in better shape for longer is to reduce this stress placed on blood vessels by lowering blood pressure. Just as when the number of heavy vehicles on main freeways is reduced, the road will last longer. In those with hypertension, for every 1mmHg decrease in systolic blood pressure, the long-term risk of a heart attack is reduced by 2 to 3 per cent.

Systolic blood pressure levels to less than 140mmHg can be achieved in most people with diabetes with regular exercise, healthy diet and medication. The benefit of targeting even lower blood pressure levels remains controversial. While it does not seem to further reduce the risk of heart attacks, the risk of stroke can be substantially reduced by lowering blood pressure below 140mmHg. This may be particularly important in women, people of an Asian background and those with atherosclerosis in the arteries that lead to the brain.

Good glucose control

In people with diabetes there is a continuous relationship between blood glucose and the risk of a heart attack. This begins around an HbA1c of 7 per cent. The higher your glucose levels above this target and the longer that this exposure occurs, the higher your risk of having a heart attack. Keeping your glucose levels under control reduces your chance of having a heart attack by at least 10 to 15 per cent. Most people with type 2 diabetes can safely achieve an HbA1c target of around 7 per cent.

The benefit of good glucose control appears to be greatest in those recently diagnosed with diabetes, in people with poor diabetes control, and before they develop heart disease. In fact, the effect of glucose control achieved in the early years after being diagnosed with diabetes has a significant influence on the subsequent risk of complications in the years following. A period of good glucose control at the start can result in a reduced risk of heart disease and other complications that persists for over a decade later, even if this good control is no longer maintained. Equally, a period of lax control at the beginning can cast a pall over your future. This is known as the **legacy effect** or **metabolic memory**.

In those who already have heart disease, the benefits of aggressively targeting lower glucose targets in terms of reducing the risk of further heart attacks or dying appears to be much smaller, or potentially not significant 'after the horse has already bolted'. However, this does not mean that glucose control has no part to play in the prevention of other complications (such as kidney and eye disease). It's just that once heart disease is established, achieving other treatment targets may reap greater rewards (such as lowering the lipid levels or blood thinners).

Stop smoking

Smoking significantly increases your risk of a heart attack as well as other complications from your diabetes. Toxins contained in cigarette smoke stress the surface of blood vessels, as well as increasing your blood pressure and cholesterol levels. Even passive smoking puts your heart at risk. So encourage your partner and your workmates to stop as well!

Stopping smoking may be one of the most important things you can do to reduce your chances of complications from type 2 diabetes.

But it's hard to do on your own. Smoking is a powerful addiction that is understandably hard to break. Like managing diabetes, the best chances of quitting for good come if you can get some help. There are lots of people and effective therapies that can help you stop smoking. Individually, they won't work the same for everyone, or in all cases. But it is usually possible to find one that will work for you. Talk to your doctor or call your local 'quit smoking line' to find out the options that best suit your needs.

One of the big concerns about stopping smoking is weight gain. Weight gain after quitting is real but it's usually small and temporary, and the health benefits of quitting more than make up for this. As you begin to feel healthier, and are able to become more active, weight levels will often return to previous levels, or lower.

The good news is that if you can quit for good, you can reverse some of the damage caused by smoking. If you can keep off the cigarettes for more than a decade your risk of heart attack and stroke are almost as low as those of a non-smoker. And there will be many other benefits along the way, so start looking at the options now.

Waist management

Waist management is a key component of diabetes management and is discussed in detail in Chapter 4. In people with type 2 diabetes, getting rid of excess fat is helpful for many reasons. One of the most important is that it can reduce the incidence and improve your outcomes from heart disease. This is achieved partly by improving risk factors for heart disease such as control of glucose, blood pressure and cholesterol levels. But over and above these gains, moderate and sustained weight loss (i.e. 7 to 10 per cent of your body weight for at least a year) will also reduce your risk of having a heart attack.

Increased physical activity

Regular physical activity has positive effects to decrease the risk of heart attacks. These include helping to maintain weight loss, improving glucose, lipid and blood pressure control, elevating mood, optimising blood flow and reducing blood clotting. These benefits are discussed in detail in Chapter 5. There are a number of different ways to stay active, from an increase in daily lifestyle activities (like walking or climbing stairs) to more structured forms of exercise in a gym. One isn't really better than another. What seems to matter is that you are regularly doing something physical, and sticking at it. Gym membership is useless if you never go. Even if you are 80 years old, starting a regular exercise routine for the first time reduces your risk of heart disease. Even if you already have diabetes, physical activity will improve your health compared to remaining on the couch. It is better late than never.

Stress management

There is no doubt that stress can be a killer. In particular, it is well known that a high level of stress is a major risk factor for heart attacks. For some people it is as important as being overweight or having high blood pressure. The stress that sets the heart pounding can come from many different sources; whether this is a major life event, job or family stress, mental, spiritual or physical stress is of less importance than its effects on you and your heart. Overall it has been estimated that up to one-third of all heart attacks may be attributable to chronic stress.

Those individuals feeling the tension of stress are at greater risk of suffering a heart attack. For example, those with persisting negative emotions (depression, anxiety or anger) have 2 or 3 times the risk of a heart attack than those without the added stress. This is partly because stress increases the work of the heart, increases the blood pressure, raises cholesterol and glucose levels, and increases blood clotting. It is also hard to focus your mind on diabetes control when your attention is stuck somewhere else.

There are many different ways to limit unwanted stresses, by augmenting resources and your ability to cope, or modulating the stress response itself. These include relaxation, hypnosis, disclosure, conditioning, avoidance and other behavioural interventions. There are also medications that can be useful in some individuals suffering from chronic stress. The most important step is identifying that stress is a problem, and getting help finding your way around it (see Chapter 16).

Thinning the blood

When a heart attack occurs, a thick clot is responsible for blocking an artery supplying the heart. Another way to reduce the chance of a major pile-up is to thin the blood, much like increasing the distance between cars on a freeway. If there is an accident it is less likely to block the whole road, and will perhaps only affect a single lane. For those at very high risk of heart disease, such as those who have previously experienced a heart attack, regularly taking drugs that slow the clotting process (such as low-dose aspirin, dipyridamole or clopidogrel) can reduce the risk of a heart attack by 20 to 25 per cent.

The use of aspirin in people who have never had a heart attack or stroke is controversial. Combined data from clinical trials suggests that aspirin has only a small or no net effect when used in all people with diabetes who don't have heart disease (i.e. a less than 10 per cent reduction in risk). But some people with diabetes have a very high risk of having a heart attack, including those with uncontrolled high blood pressure, high cholesterol levels, kidney disease, older patients, chronic smokers, and those with a strong history of heart disease in their relatives. In such cases your doctor may recommend taking low-dose aspirin (75–150mg per day). Blood thinners should not be used in people with an increased risk for bleeding, such as those who have peptic ulcers or other problems associated with intestinal bleeding and those who need to take other medications that increase the risk of bleeding, such as warfarin or anti-inflammatory drugs.

A diet rich in omega-3 fats is also associated with a reduced risk of having a heart attack, possibly because of its effects on clotting. Menaquinone (vitamin K2), which is found in green leafy vegetables and some supplements, may also have beneficial effects on clotting and may lower the risk of having a heart attack.

Don't ignore the symptoms

There are now many different ways to rapidly restore blood flow along blocked arteries following a heart attack. These are most effective when delivered as close to the first moment of blockage as possible. The longer arterial blockage is left, the greater the damage to the heart and the more limited any recovery. Time is (heart) muscle.

If you or your doctor calculate that you are at risk of having a heart attack, it is imperative you are familiar with the warning signs of a heart attack, and have an action plan for what to do in an emergency and when to call for an ambulance.

It is always better to be proactive and report any sudden new symptoms rather than hope they will go away. This may be more lifesaving than any other intervention in diabetes. The symptoms of a heart attack may include:

» sudden tightness, pressure or (crushing) pain in the chest that spreads to the shoulder, arm or jaw and doesn't go away

» suddenly feeling short of breath, nauseous, sweaty or faint for no reason (even in the absence of any pain).

It is not unusual for people with diabetes to suffer a heart attack without experiencing any symptoms (known as a **silent myocardial infarction**). This is because the nerves that supply the heart may be damaged by diabetes and are therefore unable to transmit the signals of pain through to your brain. This is why any unusual symptoms should be investigated in anyone with diabetes at risk of heart disease.

Screening for damage

If you are experiencing chest pain with exertion or other symptoms suggestive of heart problems, your doctor will often arrange additional tests to determine how well your coronary arteries are functioning, to identify the earliest signs of problems, and to direct the type and intensity of future treatments. Some of these tests may include:

» *Exercise stress testing.* You will be asked to pedal an exercise bike or walk on a treadmill to get your heart working hard. At the same time the health of your heart will be monitored by electrodes placed on the skin over your heart and on your arms. If the heart shows signs of stress with this workload, this is taken as a sign that the blood supply to the heart is not what it should be and further investigations are necessary.

» *Dobutamine stress test.* Instead of pedalling to get your heart working, in this test a chemical (dobutamine) is infused into your body to get the heart working hard. At the same time the health of your heart will be monitored by an ultrasound machine (known as an **echocardiogram**) or nuclear perfusion imaging (known as single photon emission computed tomography or SPECT scanning for short). Again, if the heart shows signs of stress with a workload, then this is taken as a sign that the blood supply to the heart is not what it should be and further investigations are necessary.

While symptoms are a reliable indicator of heart disease, typical symptoms are often masked in people with diabetes (known as **silent ischaemia**), especially those with advanced age or who are very overweight, and those with other complications affecting the eyes/kidneys or sensation in the feet. In such circumstances your doctor may also sometimes order these tests of your coronary arteries to be sure that nothing important is missed. Such testing may also be important before embarking on a program of vigorous exercise.

Road works are sometimes necessary

If the damage to the road becomes dangerous to vehicles, sometimes road works may be necessary. If you have severe damage to your blood vessels, each of these procedures can be lifesaving and life-prolonging. Such work may include scraping out any narrowing (known as **endarterectomy**) or making the road wider (known as **angioplasty**) and holding it open with a metal **stent**, or even building a bypass around the damaged area (known as **coronary artery bypass grafting** or **coronary surgery**). There is some data to suggest that early coronary surgery may be the preferred therapy in patients with diabetes when road works are required, especially using the internal mammary artery. However, such surgical interventions are also associated with significant health risks that are also greater in those with diabetes. So a balance between risks and benefits must always be struck between you and your cardiologist regarding what is the best approach for your specific problems.

Heart failure and diabetes

Any damage to the heart has the potential to reduce its ability to pump blood around the body. This is known as **heart failure**. It commonly follows a heart attack. To maintain the same output after a heart attack, the rest of the heart must work harder and faster.

To try to compensate, the pressure of fluid returning to the heart also increases to make the heart fill better. This is the equivalent of a 'head of steam' in an engine. This backup of fluid from the heart results in a number of signs and symptoms of heart failure, including the following:

» You may experience **shortness of breath**, particularly on exertion, as the ability of the heart to step up a gear is limited.

» You may also feel **short of breath when lying down**. This is because when you lie down more blood is able to return to the heart instead of pooling in your legs due to gravity. This means more work for it to do. And if the functions of the heart are impaired there will be a greater backup of fluid into your lungs, which affects your breathing.

» You might get swollen feet and lower legs (known as **oedema**) as more fluid backs up from the heart.

» Heart failure also results in the chambers of the heart becoming stretched and dilated. This can trigger irregular heartbeats or change the rhythmical beating of the heart (known as **arrhythmias**). These may be experienced as palpitations or dizzy spells.

» Eventually these compensations can no longer keep the heart pumping strongly, and as the output of blood from the heart falls, so does the blood pressure.

People with type 2 diabetes are unusually prone to heart failure; it is four- to fivefold higher in someone with diabetes than in someone without it. This is partly because heart attacks are more common, and are often recognised late in those with diabetes. However, beyond coronary artery disease, diabetes can also have direct effects to reduce the function of the heart muscle to contract and relax properly (known as **diabetic cardiomyopathy**). For example, with long-standing diabetes and high blood pressure the heart can become stiffer. A stiffer, or non-compliant, heart can't fill with blood very easily (known as **diastolic dysfunction**). So to make sure it keeps filling and pumping, the pressure inside the heart must rise; in essence, force-filling the stiff heart with blood. This also leads to shortness of breath, particularly on exertion, as the time available to fill the heart is shorter the faster the heart is beating, so that heart stiffening becomes the limiting factor.

Another feature of the heart in diabetes is that there is often damage to the nerves that are required to carefully regulate its functions. Approximately one-third of people with type 2 diabetes will have damage to the nerves that supply the heart. This damage can sometimes lead to unresponsive and/or unbalanced electrical activity. For example, when you exercise, your heart beats faster to cope with the extra demands of pushing blood to and from the exercising muscles. But if the nerves that relay these signals are damaged, the heart doesn't respond, so you stay stuck in first gear. This can also sometimes mean you don't have the energy to exercise, or that your heart stays fast all the time. Another symptom may be feeling dizzy, lightheaded or faint when standing up too quickly or when standing for too long (known as **orthostatic hypotension**).

Your heart will go on

It is hard to think about type 2 diabetes without also thinking about heart disease. It is very easy to become frightened. It is also easy to want to give up. But the heart is a surprisingly resilient organ. It has the capacity to compensate against all manner of calamities to keep the blood pumping. To some extent it even has the capacity for regeneration. There really are second chances in life.

For many people with type 2 diabetes this comes after their first heart attack, when things really hit home. But even after this kind of damage, your heart has the capacity to adapt and even improve its function. With time, the damaged area of the heart contracts to become a scar while the remainder of the heart expands to take over the work of the piece that has been lost. This is the time when other changes can also be made in your diet and lifestyle, and the targets for your treatment revised. For example, rather than stopping you in your tracks there is good evidence to show that appropriate exercise training after a heart attack can help the heart recover and keep it safe for the future. This is best conducted as part of a total program known as **cardiac rehabilitation**.

Although rehabilitation is still possible after a heart attack, taking steps to get your risk factors under control will work even better without having had the heart attack in the first place. The changes of atherosclerosis that lead to heart attacks are reversible. The instability that ultimately leads to erosions in the surface of blood vessels is reversible. And the plan of diabetes management is to do all that is possible to reverse them.

11.
Diabetes in my sight

UNDERSTAND

» The tissues of the eye are uniquely vulnerable to the effects of diabetes. It is normal for most people with type 2 diabetes to have some changes in their eyes.

» Of all the complications of diabetes, those that affect the eyes appear to be the most preventable through good diabetes management. A combination of good metabolic control, regular screening and vigilant management may reduce the risk of serious eye problems by more than two-thirds.

» Cataracts are 2 to 5 times more common in people with diabetes.

» Diabetic macular oedema is the major cause of vision loss in people with type 2 diabetes.

» It's often very hard to recognise that your own vision is declining.

MANAGE

» Maintain good control of your glucose, lipid and blood pressure levels.

» Get your eyes tested regularly by an eye expert (optometrist or ophthalmologist) so that interventions to protect the retina can be instituted in a timely manner when they are likely to be most effective.

» Report any sudden changes in your vision to your doctor or eye specialist as soon as possible.

» Don't just suffer dry or itchy eyes. Talk to your doctor about treatment options including drops or changes to your medication.

Clear and comfortable vision is easy to take for granted. Whether reading or working, driving or just watching television, good eyesight is very important to allow you to do the things you want to do. One of the things that most people know about type 2 diabetes is that it can affect your eyesight.

Diabetes is certainly a major cause of blindness in adults. However, diabetes seldom means going completely blind. Although this can rarely happen, the effects of diabetes on vision are usually more subtle. Rather than blocking an image entirely,

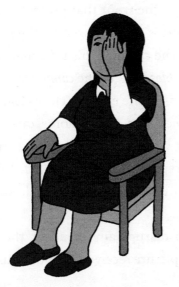

One of the things that most people know about type 2 diabetes is that it can affect your eyesight. Yet of all the complications of diabetes, those that affect the eye are the most preventable.

diabetes more commonly reduces its qualities — its colour, its detail (contrast) and/or its sharpness (focus).

While the tissues of the eye are vulnerable to the effects of diabetes, at the same time, of all the complications of diabetes those that affect the eye appear to be the most preventable by good diabetes management.

A combination of good metabolic control, regular screening and vigilant management may reduce the risk of serious eye problems by more than two-thirds. Today, most people with type 2 diabetes retain excellent vision.

How does diabetes affect your eyes?

To understand what diabetes can do to your eyes, it is first important to understand how the many different components of the eye contribute to your vision.

At its most basic, the eye works just like a digital camera. To get a clear image into your computer's memory (your brain), requires a number of steps. To take a clear photo with a camera, light must pass through the glass at the front that protects the inner workings of the camera. Light is then focused by the *lens* onto digital *sensors* at the back of the camera. This information is then packaged and relayed via *cables* back to the *computer*.

Roughly the same thing happens in the eye. For clear vision, light must pass through the *cornea*, the glassy dome on the front surface of the eye. It must be focused by the *lens*, and then activate the sensor (photoreceptor) cells of the *retina*. This information is then packaged and relayed via *nerves* back into the *brain* (computer).

Diabetes has the potential to disrupt any or all of these components and, with it, spoil the picture received by your brain.

Diabetes and the cornea

At the very front of the eye is a clear, glassy layer known as the **cornea**. This is just like the protective glass that covers the lens and workings of a camera. For the eye to work, this layer must be kept clean. Any smudges on the surface have the potential to distort images that reach the back of the eye. Diabetes can sometimes affect the functions of the cornea (known as **keratopathy**).

Because your soft eye sticks out into the world, the front of the eye is normally very good at protecting itself from damage. A healthy eye is exquisitely sensitive to even the smallest speck of dust or a misplaced eyelash, causing you to tear up and blink rapidly until the irritation is cleared away. Diabetes often damages the nerves whose job it is to sense things that might be damaging. The same changes that lead to numbness in the feet (see Chapter 12) can also reduce the sensitivity of the eye to things that might damage it. And just like the feet, the cornea of people with diabetes is more prone to scratches, ulcers and infection. The cornea can also become thicker in people with type 2 diabetes, just like calluses on your feet that result from excessive pressure and repeated injury. At the same time, healing of the cornea may be slow in people with type 2 diabetes. This can represent a major problem after cataract surgery (see below).

Another complication of diabetes is **dry eye syndrome**. As the name suggests, this results in your eyes becoming dry and easily irritated, making them feel itchy and burning, and more prone to becoming bloodshot. It can also make it hard to concentrate when reading, working or driving. This is a common problem in all adults as they age, especially women, but it is more common in people with type 2 diabetes. Tears normally form a thin film over the surface of the eye to protect the cornea from damage. Tear production lessens with age, and diabetes leads to a further reduction in the production and quality of tears, which makes dry eyes more likely. Certain medications used by people with diabetes (such as antidepressants, diuretics and some painkillers) also make dry eye more likely. But you don't have to put up with it. Dry eye can be treated using eye drops (lubricants).

Diabetes and the aqueous humour

Between the cornea and the lens sits a thin layer of clear fluid, known as the **aqueous humour** (which is more like jelly than aqueous water). It is not merely a space-filler but plays an important role in maintaining the health of the eye. Its fluids provide nutrients and other useful things (such as antibodies and antioxidants) to the clear parts of the eye, where no blood vessels can go (otherwise they would get in the way of light and obstruct your vision).

This part of the eye also maintains the (low) pressure of the eyeball (of around 10–20mmHg), which ensures blood can flow freely into the eye. If pressure in the eye rises above this level, like pumping air into a balloon, it becomes harder and harder to fill and supply the eye with the factors it needs to remain healthy. Most vulnerable to any increase in pressure are the delicate nerves that relay signals from the retina to the brain. If pressure should rise in the eye, these nerves are the first to be damaged. This is known as **glaucoma**.

The most important risk factor for glaucoma is age. It is much more common in older people than younger ones. Glaucoma is also more commonly seen in women and in people with high blood pressure, migraine, short-sightedness or a family history of glaucoma. Diabetes may also increase the risk of glaucoma by damaging the blood vessels in the coloured portion of the eye (known as the iris) that control the drainage of aqueous humour from the eye and ultimately the pressure within the eyeball.

Glaucoma is usually painless. Nerve damage usually starts very gradually in the far corners of your eyesight (eventually producing what is known as **tunnel vision**). However, vision loss gradually works its way inward so that, like a silent thief, eventually all vision is ultimately lost without treatment. Rarely, glaucoma can appear suddenly and painfully, if the outflow of the fluid from the eye is suddenly obstructed and pressure in the eyeball rapidly rises (known as **closed angle glaucoma**).

There are no simple ways to prevent glaucoma. However, it is possible for your eye specialist to detect raised pressure (greater than 20mmHg) in the eyeball using tonometry (see below). Sometimes characteristic changes of glaucoma can be seen in the back of the eye during a routine examination. If glaucoma is detected early enough, it is possible to slow its progression using eye drops (to reduce the production of aqueous humour and the pressure inside the eyeball) and pills. Laser treatments or surgery are sometimes also required to create a new passage for fluid to drain from the eye (known as **trabeculoplasty**).

Diabetes and the lens

Diabetes can also affect the lens in the eye. The lens sits in the middle of the eye and is about 1cm (⅓in) in diameter. The job of the lens is to focus light coming into the eye by changing its shape/curvature (known as **accommodation**) so that any image that reaches the back of the eye is sharply defined with clear edges and contrast. When looking into the distance, the lens becomes long and flat. But when looking at objects close up, such as when reading or sewing, the lens must retract to become smaller and rounder to accurately focus the incoming light onto the retina.

Many people with type 2 diabetes experience blurring of their vision and/or difficulty in reading when their glucose control gets either better or worse. Often blurred vision is the first symptom of diabetes. This is not due to eye damage. In fact, these symptoms usually last only a month or two and settle once glucose levels are stable again. It is caused by changes in the focusing power of the lens, as the amount of stored sugars in the lens becomes mismatched with the amount of glucose in your blood. Although you might think you need a new pair of glasses, and these could help you to see for a short while, after a month or two you'll need a new prescription as your lens returns to balance. This is why it is recommended that you should only get glasses fitted when your glucose control is stable. Otherwise further changes in your glasses prescription may be needed.

A healthy lens is normally very elastic, allowing it to quickly and efficiently change shape. But with age the lens becomes progressively stiffer. And stiff lenses simply cannot easily change shape. This means the ability of the eye to focus on nearby objects also becomes progressively reduced (known as **short-sightedness** or **presbyopia**). Everyone will eventually have this problem to some extent as they get older.

Diabetes also makes the lens less flexible. So when ageing and diabetes combine, the result can be a more rapid decline in vision and/or problems beginning at a younger age.

This progressive stiffening of the lens is a very slow process, so it may be hard to notice it yourself — sometimes it's only when people realise they are holding reading materials further and further away from them in order to focus. This is colloquially known as the 'short arm syndrome'. This is because, although holding books a little further away helps for a while, as the lens becomes stiffer you'll always need to hold things just a little bit further away. Eventually, your arms become 'too short' and some extra help is needed to focus on things close-up.

Lens stiffening does not always result in poor close-up vision. In some people, eyesight is maintained or may even improve as they get older (known as **second sight**). However, this does not mean that lens stiffening has not occurred. There's usually another factor at work, like being short-sighted to begin with, which means that instead of putting glasses on to read you now have to take your (distance) glasses off to see.

The most common treatment options for short-sightedness are to wear reading glasses, bifocals or contact lenses. Each of these treatments has its advantages and disadvantages, and is really a matter of individual preference. A number of new techniques have also been developed which can improve eyesight and help you avoid glasses or contacts. These are collectively known as **refractive surgery** and include surgically replacing the damaged lens, as well as newer techniques like inlays and laser therapy. The most common form of refractive surgery is known as **monovision**, where one eye is corrected for reading and other close-up work and the other eye is left to see things clearly in the distance. This can work quite well, but it does not work for everyone. Some people can feel uncomfortable with the changes in their vision as a result of this procedure.

The same changes that make the lens stiffer can also make the lens less transparent. This is known as a **cataract**. Cataracts are very common in everyone as they get older. At least half of all people will experience a degree of vision loss due to cataracts at some time in their life. But again, diabetes acts to speed up this process and increase its severity, so that cataracts are 2 to 5 times more common in people with type 2 diabetes.

Most cataracts are small and cause no or few symptoms like short-sightedness. They are often incidentally detected during routine eye examinations. Other early symptoms of a cataract may include things appearing less vivid with less contrast, especially in low light, as the cataract scatters the light entering your eye. Some people with cataracts also have difficulty telling colours apart, like blue and green, or may experience glare with bright lights, such as when driving at night. Eventually, cataracts can obstruct the passage of light into the eye and block your vision. Typically both eyes are affected, but usually one side is worse than the other.

Apart from age and diabetes, other factors also make cataracts more likely including cigarette smoking, excessive alcohol use, the use of steroids (as tablets but not as an inhaler for asthma) and excessive exposure to ultraviolet light (from sunshine or tanning lamps). Consequently, wearing sunglasses, wearing a brimmed hat and avoiding direct sunlight during the peak hours of ultraviolet radiation are important ways to reduce your risk of future cataracts, as well as other problems, such as skin cancer and wrinkles.

There are no medications or supplements that are able to prevent cataracts. Good diabetes control is able to modestly reduce your likelihood of developing cataracts, but will not completely prevent them.

Surgery is currently the only cure for cataracts. The good news is that cataract surgery can restore working vision in most cases if it should ever get that bad. The procedure is relatively simple and is done one eye at a time. The most common form of surgery removes the damaged part of the lens (known as **lens extraction**) and replaces it with a synthetic substitute. However, synthetic lenses are not as flexible as a healthy human lens, so they tend to provide good vision only for either distance or close up, but not both. It is usually still necessary to use reading glasses for close work (or distance glasses to focus in the distance). Cataract surgery in people with diabetes can also increase the risk of macular oedema (a serious eye problem detailed later in this chapter). This means that your eyes must be very closely monitored if you have just had cataract surgery and treated pre-emptively with lasers at the first sign of trouble.

Diabetes and the retina

At the back of the eye there is a complex layer of sensor cells whose job it is to detect minute changes in the intensity and/or colour of light. This layer is called the **retina** and is the equivalent of film in a camera. This information is then transmitted to other cells in the retina, encoded (packaged) and then relayed back to the brain via nerve fibres which, in effect, connect the camera to the computer.

There are two main types of sensor cells, known as **rod cells** and **cone cells** because of their unique shapes. Each eye contains over 100 million rod cells, whose job it is to work in low light, to tell the difference between light and dark. They are very sensitive to light, so don't provide much help to your vision during the day. But at night or in dim light, these rod cells are the most important in determining whether or not you can see.

There are also about 7 million cone cells in each eye. The cones respond to bright daylight and take care of high-resolution colour vision. But unlike the rods, they are not sensitive enough to work in the dark. This is why things look almost black and white at night. However, the amount of light in most homes means that both rods and cones contribute to what you are able to see at night-time. There are blue, green and red cones which are each sensitive to light at different wavelengths. If you are born missing one of these types of cells, you are **colour blind**.

Different parts of the retina have different functions because of the make-up of rod and cone cells and their density of packing. In the middle of the retina where light is most focused (known as the **fovea**), cone cells that specialise in sharp detail and colour are densely packed in a hexagonal mosaic pattern, very much like a honeycomb. If diabetes damages these cone-rich parts of the eye or scatters the light reaching the centre, then one of the earliest signs is a reduction in colour vision or discrimination between colours.

The further out you go from the centre of the eye, the less dense the sensor cells are packed and the more the rod cells, which specialise in detecting small amounts of light under low light conditions, become the dominant type of cell. Damage to these areas will therefore preferentially affect your night vision.

The health of the retina is determined by the capacity of the small blood vessels in the eye to supply enough nutrients and oxygen for cells to survive. Type 2 diabetes is able to progressively damage these tiny blood vessels. These changes can be observed when looking into the eye. For example:

» Weakened walls of blood vessels can balloon out (to form **microaneurysms**).

» Weakened blood vessels can leak fat and fluid. These can look like tiny white flecks in the back of the eye (known as **hard exudates**).

» Damaged vessels are also very fragile and prone to bleed spontaneously (known as a **blot haemorrhage**).

» Damaged blood vessels also mean a reduced supply of oxygen and nutrients to parts of the retina (known as **ischaemia**). This can also disrupt the flow of nutrients along the nerves, which instead can build up and look like tiny wads of cotton wool in the retina (and are appropriately known as **cotton wool spots**).

Even with the best glucose control, it is normal for most people with type 2 diabetes to develop a small number of haemorrhages, exudates, spots and/or aneurysms in their retina (cumulatively known as **background retinopathy**).

The longer you have had diabetes, the more likely that some changes will be seen in the retina.

In general, these 'background' changes do not interfere with vision unless they become concentrated around the macula, where sensory cells are most densely packed. This may lead to swelling of the retina (known as **diabetic macular oedema** or **DME**), which can have serious consequences for eyesight. In fact, macular oedema is the most frequent cause of vision loss in people with diabetes. Without treatment approximately half of those who develop macular oedema will go on to lose at least two lines of reading on a chart over the next two years.

Since the macula is densely packed with cone cells, which provide fine detail and colour sensitivity, people with macular oedema may experience blurring of both distant and close-up vision, as well as difficulties in telling the difference between some colours. Although vision loss may appear to be rapid in those experiencing macular oedema, the processes that lead to macular oedema and vision loss are relatively slow and are often not perceptible until the very centre of the vision is itself affected at the fovea. Consequently, regular comprehensive eye examinations are important for the prevention of vision loss, so that interventions to protect the retina can be instituted in a timely manner when they are likely to be most effective. Some of these treatments may include:

» *Focal laser treatment,* where a laser beam is fired to help get rid of excess fluid or destroy unhealthy areas that promote the growth of new blood vessels. While this can slow vision loss, it rarely provides significant improvement to eyesight.

» *Surgery,* where part of the gel of the eye is removed and replaced with clear fluid. This is generally reserved for those with severe haemorrhages or detachment that threatens the macula.

» *Injections with selective antibodies* that block the growth of new blood vessels which leak fluid into the retina.

» *Injections of steroids into the eye* that reduce leakage from damaged vessels. Although effective, this treatment may be associated with an increased risk of cataracts and raised pressure in the eyeball (see above).

When damaged blood vessels become blocked, this sometimes also triggers the growth of new blood vessels in the eye (known as **neovascularisation**) in an attempt to bypass the blockage and restore the flow of oxygen and nutrients. But far from being helpful, these new vessels promote scarring and even more damage to the retina (known as **proliferative retinopathy**). As scar tissue associated with new vessels shrinks, it can sometimes pull and distort the retina, cause swelling (oedema) or, rarely, pull it right off the eyeball (known as **detachment**). These new vessels are also very fragile and prone to bleed spontaneously (or haemorrhage). This can sometimes lead to the appearance of dark spots in your vision, as clots in the retina block the light coming into the retina. Bleeding into the eye itself (known as a **vitreal haemorrhage**) can give the appearance of floating lines or webs. Very rarely, bleeding is so significant as to obstruct most of the light entering the eye, like a shade in front of your vision, so that only the difference between light and dark may be seen by the affected eye. For anyone with diabetes, these kinds of sudden changes in vision constitute a real medical emergency. Seeing your doctor or eye specialist cannot be put off until tomorrow.

The appearance of new blood vessels in the eye is also commonly managed by laser treatment, in which the unhealthy areas that promote their growth are cauterised using a high intensity beam of light. Typically, over a thousand tiny burns are made across the retina. This is generally not painful, although some people may experience discomfort which can be lessened with an injection of anaesthetic behind the eye.

The new vessels themselves are not targeted by the laser. Rather, the energy hungry rods and cones are destroyed, meaning there is more oxygen to go round and the signals to make new blood vessels are reduced. Without these signals, any new blood vessels stop growing and often partly or completely disappear. However, because the laser destroys some of the rod and cone cells, which detect incoming light in the eye, some loss of vision can occur with widespread treatment. For example, some people who have had laser therapy to their eyes complain of reduced peripheral vision, impaired night vision and/or lower contrast in their eyesight.

Rarely, the growth of new vessels continues despite laser therapy. In order to prevent more severe damage, in such cases surgery may be necessary to preserve or restore vision (known as **vitrectomy**). This involves removing part of the gel of the eye and replacing it with clear fluid.

Macular degeneration

Diabetes is not the only thing that can affect the retina as you get older. One of the most common causes of declining vision is **age-related macular degeneration (AMD)**. AMD is caused by the accumulation of focal deposits (known as **drusen**) in the macula part of the retina. An in-growth of fragile blood vessels (that are also opaque) in response to the drusen further accelerates damage to the macula and ultimately leads to some loss of vision.

Again, because the macula is affected, AMD usually leads to problems in your central vision, detail, contrast and colour sensitivity. It does not lead to total blindness, as the macula only comprises a small part of the retina and the remaining (peripheral) retina remains unaffected. Usually, enough peripheral vision remains for you to see, so people often just dismiss AMD as a 'touch of old age'. But the loss of central vision can have a major effect on your functioning. For example, it may not be possible to read or recognise faces without central vision, although you will see they are there.

There are several risk factors for the development and progression of AMD. The most important is age. Around one-third of octogenarians have AMD. However, obesity, smoking, high blood pressure and high cholesterol levels also make AMD more likely as you age.

Although diabetes does not cause AMD directly, AMD is more common in people with type 2 diabetes because they are often overweight and have increased levels of blood pressure and cholesterol.

There is also some evidence that vision declines earlier and faster in people with AMD and type 2 diabetes than in those without diabetes.

The current treatment for macular degeneration involves laser therapy, although new options are being increasingly explored, including injections with selective antibodies or drugs that block the growth of new blood vessels. While these treatments may prevent further vision loss, at present no treatment is able to restore damaged nerves to the eye or improve eyesight once lost.

Preventing eye damage in diabetes

Many of the things you are already doing as part of your routine diabetes management will be improving the health of your eyes, as well of other aspects of your health. There is good evidence that the techniques to control blood glucose levels and optimise lipid and blood pressure levels will reduce the risk of developing eye problems associated with diabetes. Some blood pressure-lowering drugs such as ACE inhibitors and angiotensin-receptor blockers may have additional advantages for preventing eye damage over other drugs (see Chapter 6). But even when you are on the right medications, and your glucose, lipids and other risk factors for eye problems are under control, it is still possible for diabetes to affect your eyes. This is why everyone with type 2 diabetes should get their eyes checked on a regular basis.

Regular eye examinations

It's often hard to recognise that your own vision is declining. This is why regular testing of your vision is an extremely important part of routine diabetes management.

Getting your eyes examined regularly by an eye expert (an optometrist or ophthalmologist) is the most important thing you can do to protect your eyesight. Don't wait until you notice problems with your vision. In diabetes, the damage to your eyes is insidious. There is no pain and few symptoms.

An eye examination should be done at least every year in people with type 2 diabetes, even if their vision is normal. Eye examinations will need to be performed more frequently if you have an increased risk of eye complications (e.g. if you already have early signs of damage, high blood pressure or kidney disease). An eye examination is a simple, painless procedure that is performed by your eye care specialist. A complete eye check-up may include:

» Examining the back of your eye (the retina). To do this, your pupils may need to be dilated with eye drops so that the entire retina can be examined in detail and sometimes photographed, to allow easy comparison with previous results. These drops can sometimes make your vision blurry for a short time, so don't drive from your appointment. Dilated pupils also make you more sensitive to bright light. This can be prevented by briefly wearing your sunglasses.

» Testing your visual acuity (e.g. letter charts).

» Testing the coordinated movement of your eyes in all directions (e.g. following a light).

» Cataract evaluation (e.g. shining a light into your eye and observing the 'red eye' reflection light bouncing off your retina).

» Testing the pressure in your eyeball (known as **tonometry**) to check for early signs of glaucoma).

» Checking your colour and night vision with special charts.

» Checking the health of the macula using an Amsler grid test. This involves staring at a black dot which sits inside a grid of intersecting lines. In healthy vision, all the lines around the dot will look straight and evenly spaced. If the lines appear bent, distorted or missing, then the macula is not doing its job.

Although most emerging problems can be picked up in a routine eye examination, sometimes things can change rapidly in your eyes. If this should ever happen, it is very important to report any sudden changes in your vision to your doctor or eye specialist as soon as possible. The early detection of sight-threatening changes in your eyes is very important, because it usually allows something to be done about it. There are a number of effective treatments for eye damage that are able to help preserve your eyesight. These treatments are most effective when damage is caught in its early stages. Don't ever shut your eyes to problems with your diabetes.

12.
Diabetes on my feet

» Changes in your feet are a common complication of longstanding type 2 diabetes, reflecting a reduced ability to heal combined with an increased propensity to become damaged.

» Foot ulcers precede at least eight out of every ten lower limb amputations in people with type 2 diabetes, so are worth preventing.

» Diabetes slowly causes damage to the nerves supplying the feet and lower legs, making them numb to injury, damaging pressure or rubbing from footwear.

» Damage to the nerves may also make the muscles in the foot weak or uncoordinated which can lead to deformities such as bunions, hammer toes or claw toes.

» Serious foot problems don't occur in everyone with diabetes, but extra special care should be taken in those people at high risk of developing a foot ulcer.

MANAGE

» Control glucose, lipids and blood pressure, and stop smoking to reduce your risk of complications from diabetes in your feet and everywhere else.

» Understand your personal risk for foot problems from diabetes, and the intensity with which you need to protect your feet.

» Don't go barefoot. Without sensation you can't always rely on your feet to tell you when they are in harm's way.

» Report any changes in your feet to your doctor or foot specialist as soon as they are identified. Don't ignore them and hope they will go away by themselves. Certainly don't try to treat them yourself.

» Take care of your toenails or get someone to do this for you.

Diabetes is important everywhere in the human body and nowhere more so than in your feet. While much is made of the amorous heart and the more glamorous brain, what gets you where you need to go is your connection with your feet. Looking after this part of your health can keep you mobile, independent and on your toes.

Foot care is a key component of all diabetes management.

Changes in your feet are a common complication of type 2 diabetes. They reflect a reduced ability to heal, combined with an increased tendency to get damaged. The most dangerous changes result from a breakdown in the barrier formed by the skin, letting the dirty outside world under your skin and into your body. These may include cracks, fissures and **foot ulcers** (where the skin is completely lost over one particular area). One in seven adults with type 2 diabetes will develop a foot ulcer during their lifetime.

Preventing foot ulcers is a top priority. This is because at least eight out of every ten lower limb amputations in people with type 2 diabetes start off with a foot ulcer. However, most foot ulcers are preventable by meticulous care of your feet.

When identified and treated early, most foot complications are also manageable.

Why does diabetes damage your feet?

Diabetes can make it more likely that you get foot ulcers and other foot complications in a number of different ways (usually in disastrous combination).

Diabetes slowly causes damage to the nerves supplying the feet and lower legs (known as **neuropathy**). This can make them numb to injury, damaging pressure or rubbing from footwear (known as loss of **'protective' sensation**). Nerve damage usually goes undetected, as it's hard to be aware of what you can't feel. However, some people experience numbness in their feet, as if wearing 'socks' or 'stockings'. Nerve damage can also sometimes be painful, producing a 'pins and needles' or burning sensation in your feet, which is often worse at night.

Looking after your feet can keep you mobile, independent and on your toes. Most foot problems are very preventable.

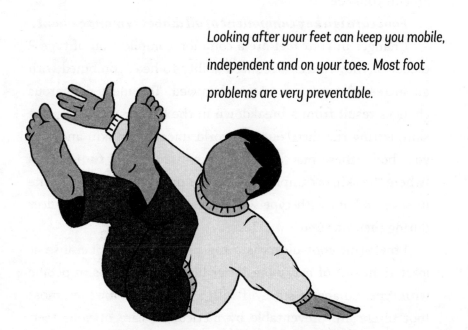

The presence of significant nerve damage may be identified by your doctor using simple clinical tools to examine if your feet can feel them or not:

» a small filament or wire may be used to test your sense of light touch

» a tuning fork may be used to test your sense of vibration

» a pin prick may be used to test your sense of sharpness

» warm and cold metal objects may be used to test your sense of cold.

A test of reflexes at the ankles is also sometimes performed. This is done by lightly striking the back of your ankle with a rubber hammer and seeing how the foot moves in response.

Some or all of these tests should be performed annually in people with type 2 diabetes to identify those who have lost their 'protective sensation', in whom a more meticulous program of foot care should be arranged (detailed later in this chapter).

Damage to the nerves may also make the muscles in the foot weak or uncoordinated. This can lead to bunions, hammer toes, claw toes or other changes in the shape of your feet (collectively known as **deformities**). These deformities create unnatural stresses and pressures on your feet, especially as your feet now don't fit into your shoes in quite the same way they used to. The extra pressure that arises from deformities can lead to skin thickening on the foot and cause corns and calluses, as well as blisters. Each is a sign that this area of the foot is being exposed to extra pressure. Overall, having a foot deformity increases your risk of getting a foot ulcer by at least threefold. In fact, most foot ulcers occur under or around these (under pressure) areas.

Diabetes can also damage both the small and large blood vessels that supply the feet, reducing the flow of blood, oxygen and sustaining nutrients to what is the furthest reach of your circulation. This is sometimes experienced as intermittent pain in the legs when walking (known as **claudication**) which is relieved by resting or elevating your feet. However, many people (possibly the majority) with poor circulation will not have any pain, especially if nerve damage is also present. The first sign may be a foot ulcer. Poor circulation can sometimes be detected by your doctor if they are unable to feel pulses in the feet or ankles, or hear blood flow in your feet using an ultrasound (Doppler) test.

Swelling of your feet (known as **oedema**) is sometimes seen in people with diabetes, especially those with kidney or heart problems, as well as those using some blood pressure-lowering medications. This makes your feet larger and tighter in your shoes (causing more rubbing and increasing the chances of getting a foot ulcer); in addition, swelling can sometimes become tight enough to reduce blood flow to the feet as well as interfere with healing.

Diabetes can also change the skin covering your feet, making it thicker, drier, less resilient and more prone to blisters or cracks (especially at the heel). Nerve damage can also reduce sweating in the feet. Areas of abnormally thick, dry skin (known as **calluses**) often form over areas of your feet that are subjected to extra pressure, such as alongside the big toe or under your heel. When these areas of thick, hard skin are compressed with walking or standing, they put even more pressure on the soft tissues underneath, causing further damage.

Visual impairment associated with diabetes (see Chapter 11) also makes minor trauma to the feet more likely to occur and less likely to be recognised early.

Finally, diabetes also increases susceptibility to **infection of the skin**, by both reducing the ability to fight off bugs that get into the skin and deeper tissues through cracks or ulcers in the feet or into the toenails. Fungal infections usually start in the toenails or between the fourth and fifth toes, where the space is most compacted by pressure. These can set up local infections that, if left untreated, can spread. At its most severe, tissues in your feet can, rarely, be killed by infection (known as **gangrene**).

What should you do to protect your feet?

Many of the things you are already doing as part of your routine diabetes management will be improving the health of your feet, as well as other aspects of your health. These include optimal control of glucose, lipids and blood pressure, and smoking cessation. These are important for preventing complications of diabetes, everywhere. But it is especially the case for your feet.

Foot ulcers are not an inevitable part of diabetes. In fact, they only occur in a minority of people. This means that for most people with type 2 diabetes, nothing special is required to stay out of harm's way beyond common sense and regular assessment of the state of your feet with your diabetes care team. However, there are some people in whom foot ulcers are far more likely and for whom more can and should be done. This includes:

» people who have currently or have previously had foot problems (e.g. ulcers, calluses, deformities such as claw toes)

» people who have lost protective sensation in their feet

» people who have poor circulation to their feet

» people who have other complications from their diabetes.

Fastidious hygiene

People with type 2 diabetes who are at increased risk for foot problems should carefully wash their feet every day but not soak them or put them in hot water. Moist areas, such as between the toes, should be dried carefully to reduce the risk of maceration or infection. Antifungal powders or talc may be useful in some people to keep moist areas dry and free of infection.

Moisturise dry areas

For dry areas of skin, like the heel and the outside of the foot, there is value in keeping the skin flexible and soft to prevent cracking. This can simply be achieved by regularly applying a non-alcohol-containing moisturiser to these areas.

Safety first

Check shoes for stones, sticks and other foreign objects that might hurt your feet, every time you put on your shoes. Without sensation you can't always rely on your feet to tell you when they are in harm's way. Many ulcers come from unnecessarily going barefoot. It may be just a short dash to the clothesline, but it's simply not worth the risk if you accidently tread on something sharp. Wear water shoes at the beach.

The right shoes

Many ulcers come simply from wearing poorly fitting or worn out shoes that rub the skin or cause pressure. Those at risk of ulcers should always wear shoes that are properly fitted to the shape of their own foot. Don't just go off the shoe size; it is invariably wrong. Only if the shoe fits should you wear it. A good fitting shoe is not when your foot fills the entire space. When buying a shoe, your longest toe should be no less than 1.5cm (½in) from the end of the shoe, to provide sufficient room for the toes to move when you walk. The ball of your foot should also correspond to the widest part of the shoe. Watch out for slip-ons — they are designed to be tight on the skin and toes (so they don't slip off!). Much better are laces or Velcro straps, which can be loosened according to the needs of your feet and tend to provide more room for the toes. They can also be loosened as the day goes on and the feet swell a bit. Shoes should be bought later in the day when feet have swelled, so the shoes will definitely accommodate and fit correctly.

Speciality shoe stores are usually better equipped than discount or department stores, which have often never heard about diabetes or think that shoes are just a fashion item. Therapeutic shoes look like any other shoe from the outside, but have a number of refinements that help to keep your feet healthy. These include:

» thick cushioning cork or pre-fabricated insoles that can be customised to your feet
» extra depth (or in-depth) to give more room for your toes
» rocker soles which decrease the pressure on the ball of the foot.

Extra cushioning (known as an **orthotic** or **orthotic insert**) can be useful if you have an increased risk of foot problems. For example, if you have a callus on your foot this may be a sign of excessive pressure being placed at this point. To prevent it becoming an ulcer, **orthotics** can be made to specifically take the pressure off this area of skin.

The right socks

The right socks can also be important for keeping your skin dry and cool. Acrylic socks that are not tight/elastic and don't have rough seams can be useful for keeping the feet dry and cool. Some socks also have special padding. Always wear clean socks and throw out damaged, tight, frayed or thin, old ones.

Toenail care

Many foot problems begin in and around the toenails. This is partly because nails are hard and skin is soft. If the toes are placed under pressure, it is the skin that suffers the most. Thickened nails or sharp edges that dig in (without you feeling it) are often the opportunity infection needs to get started.

It is recommended that all people with type 2 diabetes should keep their toenails short by regularly having them trimmed, by themselves or others. This should always be straight across following the curve of your toes, but not too short to reduce the risk of in-grown nails. File any sharp edges with an emery board or nail file. Always have a podiatrist do this if you need help or are unsure, or can't see or reach the toes very well.

Keep a close eye on your feet

Inspect your feet every day for early signs of trouble or potential problem areas. Don't forget to check between your toes. Sometimes a mirror is helpful to see the entire bottom of your feet. Take off your shoes and socks at every doctor's appointment — it may only take a few seconds to give you the all-clear but it can be life-saving.

It is also very important to report any changes in your feet to your doctor or foot specialist as soon as they are identified. Don't ignore them and hope they will go away. Certainly, don't ever wait for them to become painful. Warning signs include:

» redness or skin discolouration, especially around corns or calluses
» swelling or change in the size or shape of your foot or ankle
» pain in the feet or legs at rest or while walking (but remember that you don't need to be feeling any pain for there to be a serious problem)

» blisters
» bleeding
» open sores (ulcers), no matter how small!
» hot or cold spots.

Avoid home remedies

Thinning areas of thick skin (a callus) on your feet can take the pressure off the skin that lies underneath. But this is not a task to be undertaken in your own 'bathroom surgery' or with over-the-counter 'corn cures'. Foot specialists (known as podiatrists) who have training in the management of the diabetic foot are widely available and should be used in any situation where preventive management is appropriate.

How are foot ulcers treated?

Each foot ulcer is different and will need to be assessed and managed differently depending on the depth of the wound, the presence or absence of infection and healthy blood flow. This is a complex and delicate process and is best coordinated by wound specialists, often acting as part of a multidisciplinary team involving doctors, wound management nurses, podiatrists and other allied health professionals.

All ulcers will require regular cleaning and any dead skin and foreign material removed from the wound (a process known as **debridement**). Dressings are then used to create and maintain an optimal environment for healing, as well as to protect the wound from further damage. There are many different dressings available, all of which will be appropriate to different situations, including saline, disinfectants, gels and ointments.

If you have an ulcer, your doctor will often advise you to rest and limit your walking. This is not some idle request. Staying off your feet is sometimes vital for effective healing. Continued pressure to the bed of a wound can prolong healing or sometimes result in even more damage. It may seem excessive to be on crutches, using a walker or a wheelchair for just a little ulcer, but the complications of a non-healing ulcer may be far worse.

In many cases **off-loading devices** (such as padding, therapeutic shoes, orthotics, casts, walking aids, etc.) can relieve the pressure on ulcers and help with healing while you are maintaining your regular daily activities. Some can even be taken off at night or for a bath. Their only problem is that any walking without the cast, even for a short distance, can undo all the good of having rested your foot.

Antibiotics will sometimes be used to help an infection heal and prevent it from spreading. Antibiotic cream might be placed directly on the wound, tablets might be taken or an injection given. Antibiotic therapy on its own is always insufficient to heal an ulcer. And it's important to realise you can't just use any old antiseptic cream from the bathroom cabinet to fix such foot problems — some of these may be too strong for the feet of someone with diabetes and may do more harm than good. Antibiotic treatment is usually continued until there is evidence that the infection has resolved, but not necessarily until the ulcer has healed.

Surgery is sometimes necessary to help foot ulcers heal. This includes procedures to improve your circulation or to correct deformities. Very rarely, **amputation** of part or all of the foot may be necessary to save the rest of the foot or leg from gangrene. In most cases this outcome can be prevented.

13

Diabetes in my kidneys

UNDERSTAND

» The kidneys perform many important tasks in keeping you healthy that allow your heart, brain, bone and many other parts of your body to do the jobs they are supposed to do.

» At least every second person with type 2 diabetes has kidney damage, manifested by increased amounts of albumin in the urine and/or a reduced ability to filter the blood.

» Having kidney disease puts you at increased risk of other complications from type 2 diabetes, including heart, foot and eye disease and hypoglycaemia.

» Good glucose, lipid and blood pressure control in someone with type 2 diabetes can reduce the risk of kidney problems by over half.

» Although it is possible to have dialysis or sometimes receive a new kidney, the health of such people is sadly never as good as those who have their own kidneys functioning.

MANAGE

» Achieve and maintain good glucose control to keep your kidneys functioning for longer.

» Treat high blood pressure levels and maintain

smooth control over them to protect your kidneys as much as your heart.

» Get even more serious about keeping your lipid levels under control. The most common serious complication of failing kidney function is heart disease, and this can be partly prevented by good lipid control.

» Get your kidney function checked at least annually.

» Encourage your friends and family to become organ donors. For those who develop kidney failure, this generous gift may be the gift of life.

The kidneys perform many important tasks to keep you healthy. You even have a spare one to make sure there is always enough capacity to deal with any extra demands and stand as insurance against any loss of function. In essence, good kidney function enables your heart, brain, bone and many other parts of your body to do the job they are supposed to do.

Impaired kidney function is a drag on everything else. The risks of heart, feet and eye problems, hypoglycaemia and many other complications are all increased in people with impaired kidney function.

The kidneys partly do their job by filtering the blood. Adults have about 5 litres (1⅓gal) of blood pumping around their body all the time. Every minute, about 1 litre (2pt) of this blood passes through the kidneys. Consequently, every 5 minutes all of the blood in the body has been filtered through the kidneys.

The filtered fluid then passes along a series of small tubes (or tubules) where any vital components (such as salt, water and glucose) are reabsorbed, leaving behind only waste (urine). This selective reabsorption system is so efficient that for every litre of blood that is filtered, less than a teaspoon of urine is made.

These tubules also actively secrete a number of toxins into the urine.

The kidneys' main priority is maintaining a strict balance of fluid inside the body. If only a small amount of fluid is drunk, the kidneys' priority is to keep hold of as much as possible, so urine production is reduced and the urine becomes more concentrated. Equally, if you drink a lot of fluid, the kidneys are able to release more water into the urine, which becomes lighter and more dilute. Either way, the amount of fluid in the body scarcely changes.

Often an early sign of diabetes may be passing urine more frequently, with more urgency, or having to get out of bed at night to go the toilet. This makes you thirsty and as a result you also tend to drink more. The term diabetes actually means 'siphon', because it appeared to the Ancient Greeks that water seemed to flow out as rapidly as it was poured in, like a siphon.

When glucose levels in the blood are under control, any glucose that is filtered through the kidneys is very rapidly reabsorbed by the tubules so as not to waste this very valuable source of energy. However, this capacity for reabsorption is limited. When glucose levels in the blood get any higher than 8 to 9mmol/L (144–162mg/dL), some glucose starts spilling over into the urine. This is rather like a safety valve, relieving the effects of high levels. However, when glucose spills over into the urine it also drags some water with it. So even if you are dehydrated, the urine of those with type 2 diabetes and poor glucose control can be surprisingly dilute, voluminous and frequent. The only way to keep up with extra water loss is to drink more. This is why uncontrolled diabetes is like a siphon.

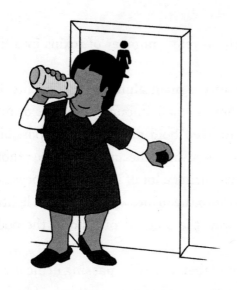

Diabetes means 'siphon', because it appeared to the Ancient Greeks that water seemed to flow out as rapidly as it was poured in!

Passing more urine is not a sign that your kidneys are damaged. In fact, it is a sign that your kidneys are doing their job. If you are able to get your glucose levels under control and maintain your glucose levels at less than 8mmol/L (144mg/dL) for most of the time, then the twin problems of passing more urine and feeling thirsty will usually settle.

How does kidney damage affect your health?

Diabetes may result in damage to many parts of the kidney. The filter units of the kidney (known as **glomeruli**) are especially vulnerable. The kidneys usually have over a million of them. They function in much the same way as a sieve: they hold onto the big things inside the blood (such as cells and big proteins) but allow the water (and any dissolved toxins) to filter down into the tubules and out into the urine. Like the damage to a sieve, damage to glomeruli can have two major effects:

»   things can get through the sieve (and end up down the drain)

»   the sieve gets clogged and it can't filter properly.

This is exactly what happens in the kidneys of people with type 2 diabetes. Firstly, instead of staying on the blood side of the filter, some proteins can leak into the urine (like pasta falling through a broken sieve and into the sink). The most common protein in your blood is **albumin**. So an early sign of kidney damage in diabetes is the presence of small amounts of albumin in your urine (known as **microalbuminuria**).

There is no pain or symptoms associated with microalbuminuria, so its detection relies on regular screening and urine testing (see below). About one-third of those with type 2 diabetes have elevated amounts of albumin in their urine. However, microalbuminuria is even more common in those who also have high glucose, high blood pressure and/or high cholesterol levels, as well those with established complications elsewhere (e.g. heart disease, eye, nerve or foot disease).

Secondly, just like a sieve, the filters of the kidney can progressively clog and become scarred, reducing the ability of your body to filter fluid and clear toxins from the blood. This is a slow process and doesn't affect all filter units all at once. But any loss means that the others have to take up the slack and work harder. This in turn causes them to burn out faster, causing more loss and more work for those remaining in a vicious circle. So by the time your kidney function becomes impaired it means that you have lost at least one kidney's worth of function. One in four people with type 2 diabetes will lose this much or more.

Although some decline in kidney function with age is inevitable, some people with type 2 diabetes are more likely to experience a more rapid fall in kidney function, including:

» people losing large amounts of albumin into their urine (as a marker of kidney disease and its severity)

» people whose blood pressure is very high and isn't easily controlled with standard medications

» people with heart disease

» people with eye problems from their diabetes

» people with foot problems from their diabetes

» people with anaemia (as a marker of kidney disease and its severity)

» people with an indigenous ethnic background

» people experiencing socioeconomic disadvantage.

As the function of the kidneys declines, to make up for any shortfall the kidneys send out signals to drive up the blood pressure. This is much like giving a car extra revs to get up a hill. The extra pressure means that more filtering can get done with fewer filters. However, this is at the expense of **hypertension**. This extra work also means they wear out faster.

One of the ways the kidneys increase **blood pressure** is by holding back more fluid from entering the urine. In addition to increasing blood pressure, this extra fluid can also lead to swelling of your legs or around your eyes (known as **oedema**). Fluid retention can also make some blood pressure-lowering medications less effective in people with impaired kidney function or increase the need for other medications that help you lose this excess fluid (known as **diuretics**).

Impaired kidney function also drives up lipid levels in the blood, which combines with high blood pressure and fluid retention to at least double the risk of heart attacks, strokes and other complications in people with type 2 diabetes who also have kidney disease.

The clearance of many medicines used to treat diabetes is also affected by impaired kidney function. Instead of being removed by the kidneys, these drugs hang around longer than they are really needed. This can sometimes mean more **side effects**. For example, the kidneys filter and remove insulin from the body. But if kidney function is impaired, insulin stays around for longer, increasing the chances it will lower glucose levels too far and cause **hypoglycaemia**. So kidney disease often means a careful reassessment of the medications you are on in order to prevent any unwanted side effects.

The kidneys do much more than just pass water (and any dissolved toxins). The kidneys also regulate the levels of calcium in your bones. Damage to your kidneys can also result in bone thinning (known as **osteoporosis**), which when combined with normal thinning with age can increase your risk of fractures.

The kidneys also regulate the level of red cells in the blood, whose job it is to carry oxygen to all parts of your body for fuel. Damage to your kidneys will therefore sometimes reduce the concentration of red cells in the blood (known as **anaemia**), which is detected by a simple blood test.

How is kidney disease detected?

Regular examination of kidney function by your doctor can help identify early signs of trouble. This should be done annually in all people with type 2 diabetes, or more often if you have increased risk of kidney complications (e.g. if you already have early signs of kidney damage, high blood pressure or eye disease). This involves two separate tests, the glomerular filtration rate (GFR) and testing the level of albumin in the urine.

The glomerular filtration rate (GFR)

The GFR is estimated on the results of a standard blood test that measures the concentration of creatinine, an abundant natural chemical that is filtered and cleared by the kidneys. As kidney function declines the level of creatinine rises in the blood. The amount by which it rises can be used to determine how far the filtration functions of the kidneys have fallen.

Albumin in the urine

The most practical test measures the amount of albumin in a urine sample from the first or second time you go to the toilet in the morning. Measurements of albumin in random urine samples (known as spot tests) are more variable and may be less accurate in determining your risks. Some doctors prefer to measure albumin in urine collected over 24 hours to document the total amount of albumin lost over the course of a day.

There is also normally substantial day-to-day variability in the amount of albumin in any one person's urine. For this reason an initial assessment of someone with type 2 diabetes will usually involve at least three urine tests taken over the first 3 to 6 months.

Once a level of microalbuminuria is established, further screening of kidney function can be undertaken annually. If normal amounts of albumin are detected at subsequent testing in someone with previously negative tests, they can simply be retested annually as part of routine assessment for complications, as it is unlikely that significant kidney problems have been missed. However, any new positive test is usually confirmed with additional tests performed during the subsequent 3 to 6 months.

How is kidney disease prevented and treated?

Although kidney damage is very common in people with diabetes, in most cases it is possible to prevent serious decline in function or complete kidney failure. All of the different aspects of diabetes care will protect your kidneys from damage, and when performed together in someone with type 2 diabetes they can reduce your risk of kidney problems by over half.

Maintaining good control of your glucose

There is a strong association between how well you are able to control your glucose levels and your risk of kidney disease.

Achieving and maintaining glycaemic targets through a combination of healthy diet, regular exercise and medication significantly reduces the chances you will develop kidney disease.

Maintaining good control of your lipids

High lipid levels are not just bad for the heart, but may be damaging to kidneys as well. Over and above their effects on heart disease, some studies have suggested that common medications used to lower lipid levels, like **statins** and **fibrates** (see Chapter 9), may also have beneficial effects on the development and progression of kidney disease.

Maintaining good control of your blood pressure

Getting your systolic blood pressure below 140mmHg is a key target for the prevention of diabetic kidney disease, as well as other complications. Although high blood pressure can be a result of kidney disease, in many cases high blood pressure may also precede the onset of kidney problems and contribute to its decline. Some blood pressure-lowering drugs such as ACE inhibitors and angiotensin-receptor blockers may have additional advantages for preventing kidney damage over other anti-hypertensive drugs. But more important is to get rid of hypertension, in whatever way this can be achieved. The use of blood pressure-lowering medication to protect the kidneys in the absence of hypertension remains controversial, including the need to push for lower blood pressure targets to protect the kidneys.

Early referral to a specialist

Sometimes, a kidney specialist can also assist in your medical care. This can be especially important for people with type 2 diabetes who have advanced kidney disease. Early planning for renal replacement, management of anaemia and other complications of failing kidney function is important. Waiting until you become unwell means that it is often harder to get your health back.

Kidney replacement

The accumulation of toxins that would otherwise be cleared by healthy kidneys can make people with severely impaired kidney function feel tired and weak, nauseous with a poor appetite, cold and itchy. Ultimately, toxins can accumulate to such an extent that a kidney transplant or some artificial means of clearing them (known as **dialysis**) is necessary in order to survive.

Diabetes is the single leading reason for needing to have dialysis and accounts for between one-third to half of all people entering dialysis programs each year. A number of different dialysis options are now available, including **haemodialysis**, where a machine filters your blood through a direct connection to your bloodstream; and **peritoneal dialysis**, where fluid is rinsed through the abdomen allowing toxins to diffuse into the fluid and then be removed as fresh fluid is replaced.

Some people with type 2 diabetes may be candidates for a kidney transplant in the event their own kidneys fail.

Transplantation involves major surgery in which a single kidney is removed from a live relative or a brain-dead organ donor who shares tissue features sufficiently similar to your own as to reduce the chances that your body will reject the new kidney (known as a match). This kidney is then connected to your blood and bladder, and will usually immediately function in filtering your blood and making urine.

Although kidney transplantation is a very effective way to save the life of people who develop kidney failure, it is not a perfect solution. There are never enough donors for everyone, and some people will wait many years on dialysis before a suitable match becomes available. By the time your kidneys fail, it is common to have many other problems with your health, including heart disease, which makes the stress of major surgery too dangerous for some people.

A number of medications are also required to prevent your body rejecting the new kidney and ensuring its survival. These can have serious side effects, including reducing your immunity, which opens the door to infection, cancer and other illnesses.

Although it is possible to have dialysis or sometimes receive a new kidney, the health of people receiving a kidney replacement is sadly never as good as those who have their own kidneys functioning. Consequently, it is much more important to protect your kidneys than to rely on modern medicine to get you out of trouble if your kidneys fail.

14.
Diabetes in my bladder

UNDERSTAND

» One sign of poor glucose control may be increased thirst along with passing urine more frequently, with more urgency, or having to get out of bed at night to go to the toilet.

» Some people with type 2 diabetes experience involuntary and inappropriate contractions of the bladder (known as an overactive bladder) that make you want to go to the toilet frequently and with great urgency.

» In other people, their bladder won't contract enough to empty fully, causing urinary retention.

» Diabetes exacerbates the urinary symptoms of pelvic floor weakness (in women) and prostatism (in men).

MANAGE

» Achieve and maintain good glucose control to slow the flow of urine, especially at night, and reduce irritability in the bladder.

» Don't suffer in silence with bladder problems. Ask your doctor for help.

» Strengthen up your pelvic floor by doing regular (Kegel) exercises.

» Establish a pattern of going to the toilet rather than being controlled by your bladder.

It is seldom appreciated by doctors that the bladder and its functions are pivotal for both productivity and quality of life. Yet this is well understood by people with type 2 diabetes, especially but not exclusively by women. Having to rush to find a toilet; having to get up many times at night; having to limit fluid intake in an attempt to stay dry — these are all common symptoms of people with type 2 diabetes if they are asked. Indeed, at least three-quarters of all people with type 2 diabetes will experience bladder problems to some degree. However, few complain without prompting, so these bothersome symptoms are seldom addressed as part of routine diabetes care. This needs to change.

About the bladder

The bladder is a balloon-shaped organ that sits in the pelvis. It coordinates two opposing functions: storing urine and peeing (voiding) it out.

As urine is made by the kidneys, it flows down the upper urinary tract into the bladder where it is stored. Although it varies from person to person, the bladder's average capacity is between 300 and 400ml (½–¾pt) before it begins to feel full. At this point, the bladder signals to the brain that it is time to urinate. These signals become more and more insistent as the volume of urine in the bladder increases.

In infants, this triggers an automatic reflex to urinate. But in adults this reflex is held in check by sheer willpower. When you reach a toilet and are fully ready to go, you consciously release this hold, the pelvic floor relaxes and the bladder contracts, allowing the urine to flow. A healthy bladder will contract fully, leaving behind only a teaspoon of urine. This cycle will be repeated on average three to four times every 24 hours, without a drop ever being spilt.

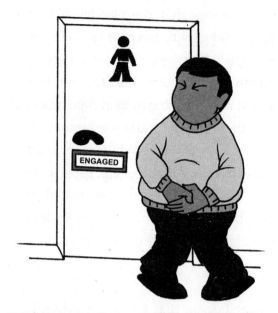

At least three-quarters of all people with type 2 diabetes will experience bladder problems to some degree.

What does diabetes do to the bladder?

Diabetes has the potential to disrupt the coordinated functions of the bladder in a number of different ways. There is often a very gradual change in toileting requirements, so people frequently overlook symptoms or put them down to just getting old. Doctors often attribute these bothersome changes to just having to pass more urine when glucose control is less than optimal.

However, just as diabetes affects the heart, the eyes and the kidneys, the same process can also disrupt the coordinated functions of the bladder. This can cause a range of different symptoms in different people.

Some people with diabetes experience involuntary and inappropriate contractions of their bladder before it is completely filled (known as **overactive bladder** or **bladder instability**). These contractions suddenly make you feel the urge to urinate (known as **urgency**), meaning you have to go to the toilet many times during the day (known as **frequency**) or have to get up many times during the night (known as **nocturia**). Sometimes you leak before you can stop it or get to a bathroom (known as **urge incontinence**).

The bladder can be jumpy like this for a number of reasons, such as if it is irritated with a bladder infection. However, diabetes itself can make the bladder more irritable, simply in response to having to deal with a greater urine output. It is thought that the bladder learns what's coming in diabetes and gets you to go sooner than would otherwise be necessary, in anticipation. This problem tends to be more common in those people who have recently been diagnosed with diabetes rather than those who have had it for many years. In other people with type 2 diabetes, their bladder may be underactive, which means it is less able to contract. This can lead to incomplete emptying of the bladder (known as **urinary retention**). The chance of still having over 100ml (3⅓fl oz) still left in your bladder after going to the toilet is at least ten times greater in those with type 2 diabetes when compared to those without diabetes. This problem tends to be more common in those who have had their diabetes for a long time rather than those who have only been recently diagnosed.

Urinary retention is often caused by nerve damage associated with diabetes that reduces the sensations the body uses to know it is time to go to the toilet. This nerve damage also disrupts the coordinated contractions that under normal circumstances empty the bladder completely each time you go.

A weak and underactive bladder may be experienced by its sufferer as a difficulty in starting to urinate or passing only a dribbling, weak stream of urine that falls off quickly. And if you can't empty your bladder fully it takes less time to be completely full again. This means you frequently have to go again and again to the toilet, through the day and night. So although your bladder may be inactive, you could be experiencing lots of bladder activity.

The longer urine is stored in the bladder, the greater the chance it will become infected, especially in women. So having urinary retention also leads to higher amounts of bacteria in the urine and a greater risk of **urinary tract infections** (known as **UTIs**).

A full bladder is also prone to unintentionally leaking small amounts of urine with coughing, exercising or other things that put stress on the bladder (this is known as **stress** or **overflow incontinence**). At least every second woman with type 2 diabetes will experience some urine leakage every month.

Women are more prone to this problem than men, due to the weakening of the pelvic floor during childbirth. The pelvic floor naturally forms a hammock across the pelvis that holds its contents in their place. During pregnancy and labour, this hammock can become stretched and weakened. At its most severe, sagging of the pelvic floor can lead to **prolapse**, when pelvic organs (the bladder, rectum or uterus) protrude into the vagina. Most women with children will have some degree of prolapse on close examination. However, very few will experience major problems as a result. But because diabetes is filling up the bladder rapidly, and increasing its volume, any symptoms of a weak pelvic floor are accentuated in women with type 2 diabetes.

What can be done about bladder problems?

Although some decline in bladder function is inevitable, there is much that can be done to keep your bladder in good shape.

» Achieving and maintaining good glucose control will slow the flow of urine, especially at night, and reduce irritability in the bladder acquired from making so much urine.

» Weight control will reduce the risk and severity of urinary incontinence in people with diabetes who are overweight.

» For a number of reasons, the most important time to look after the bladder is at night. Not only do you want a good, unbroken night's sleep, but this is the time of the day when urine output should normally slow. If it doesn't then the bladder is forced to change, making it (and you) more irritable. Simple things can be helpful, such as: keeping an eye on the amount and timing of your fluid intake; drinking most fluid in the morning or early afternoon; avoiding things that irritate the bladder like caffeine in tea and coffee; limiting alcohol intake in the evening; and fully emptying the bladder and bowels before going to bed.

Rather than suffering in silence, it is important to seek help early as many options are available to improve bladder function and quality of life. These are generally more effective the earlier they are initiated. Some of these options are examined below.

Change your behaviour

Rather than waiting for the uncontrollable urge, sometimes it is best to establish a pattern of going to the toilet frequently (every 2 to 4 hours through the day, regardless of any urge). It is also important to empty the bladder (known as **voiding**) as fully as possible each time you go to the toilet. One way to do this is the **double voiding technique**. As the name suggests, double voiding means emptying the bladder twice, by urinating a second time 10 to 15 minutes after the first time. It is a very simple way to reduce the pooling of urine in the bladder.

Pelvic floor exercises

Pelvic floor exercises are useful to strengthen the muscles of the pelvic floor which support the structures of the bladder and reduce the chance of leaking. These are also known as Kegel exercises. These exercises simply involve consciously trying to contract and relax the muscles of the pelvis, as though you want to stop a flow of urine. Hold onto the contraction for 5 seconds, then relax for 5 seconds, then repeat this ten times in a row, at least three times a day. Work your way up to keeping the muscles contracted for 10 seconds at a time, relaxing for 10 seconds between contractions. For best results, focus on tightening only your pelvic floor muscles and avoid holding your breath. Regular pelvic floor muscle training combined with bladder training can solve most bladder problems in many women. It can also be useful for men with bladder problems.

Medications for an irritable bladder

Some people with an overactive bladder can benefit from medications that reduce bladder irritability, the strength of sudden urges and the frequency of voiding. However, because of the way they work within the body, most have unwanted side effects such as dry mouth and eyes, blurred vision, sedation and constipation. Local oestrogen creams can also keep the tissues around the bladder and vagina healthy and reduce irritability in some cases.

It is often suggested that cranberry juice is good for bladder problems. However, rigorous studies do not back up these claims, and bacteria quickly become resistant to any potentially useful effects. Probiotics, such as lactobacillus in yoghurt and some supplements, are also widely touted for bladder problems, but again robust evidence for any beneficial effect is lacking.

A number of new techniques are also emerging, including electrical stimulation devices that can be used to help empty a sluggish bladder.

Surgery

Surgical treatment is sometimes necessary to fix bothersome bladder problems. This used to mean removal of the uterus, or womb (known as a hysterectomy). Although prolapse is currently the major reason for having a hysterectomy, many other options are available, especially if initiated at an early stage, including pessaries to support the pelvic floor. A number of non-destructive and less invasive surgical procedures are also now available, many with good success rates.

Diabetes and the prostate

Men also have their own special burden, the prostate gland, which sits just under the bladder. The prostate gland slowly enlarges in all men as they age, sometimes enough to slow the flow of urine. This can result in a number of troublesome symptoms including an interrupted or dribbling stream, frequency, urgency and/or incontinence. It is still controversial whether diabetes makes prostate enlargement worse. Many of the factors that lead to the development of diabetes (such as obesity, lack of physical activity, smoking and a high fat diet) are also associated with prostate enlargement. Diabetes also means that the bladder symptoms associated with prostate problems are often worse, including nocturia and urgency, which means that prostate problems may be picked up more often in men with type 2 diabetes.

Again, it is not necessary to suffer in silence or consign your symptoms to your diabetes. There are now a number of effective treatments available to get the flow going again. These include medications to shrink the prostate or relax the neck of the bladder to improve urine flow. Minimally invasive surgical options are also now available. Diets rich in phytoestrogens (found in fresh fruit, vegetables, soy, lentils, flaxseed and chickpeas), lycopenes (in red fruit such as watermelon, tomatoes), onions and garlic are also associated with lower rates of prostate enlargement, although none can fix prostate problems once they occur. Supplements containing saw palmetto extract, zinc, or beta-sitosterol are widely advertised as alternative therapies for prostate disease but have not been shown to be effective in rigorous trials. In contrast, regular exercise seems to help keep the prostate under control, as well as other parts of your diabetes management.

15

Diabetes on my mind

UNDERSTAND

» Strokes are more common in people with type 2 diabetes and their impact is greater.

» Good glucose, lipid and blood pressure control in someone with type 2 diabetes can reduce your risk of having a stroke by over two-thirds.

» Many people with type 2 diabetes will develop dementia during their lifetime. But the risk can also be reduced by good diabetes control.

MANAGE

» Become familiar with the warning signs of a stroke. Have an action plan for what to do in the event of a stroke and when to call for an ambulance.

» Achieve and maintain smooth control of your blood pressure.

The brain is central to all the functions of the body. Through the nerves and other signals, it is connected to and regulates all aspects of your health. Looking after your brain and mind is as important for managing type 2 diabetes as any other aspect of diabetes care — some would say more so. While glucose, lipid and blood pressure control are all achievable, they can seem futile when the mind is not also on board.

What are strokes and how do you avoid them?

One of the most devastating consequences of type 2 diabetes is its association with an increased risk of having a stroke. As detailed in Chapter 10, all parts of the body depend on the flow of blood for their survival. If this flow is stopped, even for a brief period, any parts downstream from the blockage suffer and may die. When a permanent blockage in blood flow to the brain occurs, it is called a **stroke** (also known as a **cerebrovascular accident** or **CVA**).

Type 2 diabetes is associated with an increased risk of strokes that is over twice that observed in people without diabetes. Approximately one in eight people with type 2 diabetes will have a stroke. The impact of having a stroke is also more serious, as the frequency of irreversible brain damage, recurrent strokes, disability and mortality are also higher in those with type 2 diabetes.

The most common cause of blockage to the blood vessels supplying your brain is **atherosclerosis**. This is the same process that leads to heart attacks (detailed in Chapter 10). In this process, increasing amounts of cholesterol are deposited in the walls of blood vessels, making them increasingly unstable and sensitive to the stresses of blood pressure. Then one fateful day there is an erosion or rupture of its protective surface and a blood vessel becomes clotted. This can be the first sign there is anything wrong.

This blockage may occur at the site of atherosclerosis or downstream of the damaged blood vessel, as bits of clot fly off only to get stuck in vessels too small to let them pass. If these blockages can't be quickly cleared, then any parts of the brain that depended on the flow of blood coming from that blood vessel will die. Unlike damage to your skin, brain cells cannot grow back, so any significant loss of flow always means some permanent loss of function.

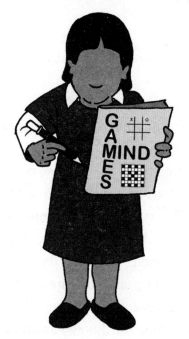

Looking after your mind is as important for managing diabetes as any other aspect of diabetes care. Some would say more so.

Age, high glucose, blood pressure and cholesterol levels, smoking and the presence of atherosclerosis elsewhere (in the heart or legs) are the major risk factors for having a stroke in a person with type 2 diabetes.

These are the same risk factors for heart disease; this is because it is essentially the same process, just in different blood vessels. Consequently, the same things that reduce the risk of heart attacks, detailed in Chapter 10, will also reduce your risk of having a stroke, including:

» reducing the systolic blood pressure and its variability
» reducing the total cholesterol levels in the blood
» raising the HDL cholesterol in the blood
» improving glucose control

» stopping smoking

» weight management

» increased physical activity

» stress management

» thinning the blood (with aspirin, dipyridamole and/or clopidogrel).

Clinical studies in people with type 2 diabetes suggest that if you do all of these things to the best of your ability, you can reduce your risk of having a stroke by over two-thirds.

Blockage of blood vessels supplying the brain may also occur if a clot forms in the heart, is dislodged and then pushed by the flow of the blood into your brain. This is known as an **embolic stroke** and is thought to account for about 10 per cent of all strokes. Clots can occur in the heart if heart valves are damaged or if the smooth flow of blood through the heart is disrupted. This can occur when some parts contract more forcefully than others or if the rhythm of the heart becomes erratic (known as **atrial fibrillation** or **AF**). This lack of coordination of the heartbeat leads to turbulence and eddies of relatively stagnant blood flow where clotting can occur. AF is more common in patients with diabetes due to their heart being stiffer (see Chapter 10). The risk of embolic stroke can be reduced in people with AF by using medication to thin the blood and prevent clotting.

Some strokes occur when there is bleeding into the brain (known as a **haemorrhagic stroke**). They result from a weakened vessel that ruptures and bleeds into the surrounding brain. The blood then accumulates and compresses the surrounding brain tissue, starving it of oxygen in essentially the same way an ischaemic stroke (see below) causes damage. Type 2 diabetes does not increase the risk of this kind of stroke, although high blood pressure, kidney disease and increasing age that accompany diabetes mean that at least 10 per cent of all strokes in those with diabetes are associated with bleeding into the brain.

As with a heart attack, all individuals with type 2 diabetes should be familiar with the warning signs of a stroke and have an action plan for what to do in the event of a stroke and when to call for an ambulance. Warning signs of a stroke may include:

» sudden weakness or heaviness of the face, arm or leg affecting only one side of the body
» sudden change in your vision, especially in one eye
» sudden change in or loss of speech, trouble talking or pronouncing words clearly or difficulty understanding them
» sudden onset of dizziness, unsteadiness or loss of balance.

There are now many different ways to rapidly restore blood flow along blocked arteries following a stroke. Again, these are most effective when delivered as close to the first moment of blockage as possible, and at the very least within 3 hours from the onset of symptoms. The longer arterial blockage is left, the greater the damage to the brain and the more limited any recovery. All those with type 2 diabetes should be proactive and report any sudden new symptoms rather than hope they will go away.

A stroke is diagnosed when someone experiences these persistent symptoms and is usually verified by a brain scan that shows reduced blood supply to one area of the brain.

Transient ischaemic attacks

Sometimes people experience only short-lived symptoms of stroke which last a few minutes but then fully resolve. This is known as a **transient ischaemic attack** or **TIA**. It is sometimes also called a mini-stroke. It represents a warning that there is something wrong with the blood vessels supplying the brain and that more serious or long-lasting damage may be just around the corner. Approximately one-third of people who experience TIA go on to have a stroke within a year.

TIAs are thought to occur when a clot blocks a damaged blood vessel to the brain, but then is quickly dissolved or is pushed away by the force of the blood pressure. Because TIAs can be a harbinger of more serious problems to come, such episodes are treated very seriously, usually with your doctor prescribing blood thinners and aiming for more intensive lipid and blood pressure control. Surgery to clean out damaged and narrowed blood vessels (known as an **endarterectomy**) may also be appropriate for people with atherosclerosis in the blood vessels of the neck that supply the brain (known as the **carotid arteries**). Doctors sometimes also recommend a balloon to dilate blocked or damaged blood vessels (known as **angioplasty**) and implantable steel screens (known as **stents**) to hold open blood vessels.

What is dementia? How do you keep your mind sharp?

For many people, one of their greatest fears is that they will experience a decline in their ability to think, remember, calculate and learn (known as **cognitive function**). Sadly, in some people these deficits can be severe and widespread, and compromise their ability to function independently; this is known as **dementia**. At least one-quarter of those with type 2 diabetes aged over 60 will develop dementia during their lifetime. Many others will suffer lesser degrees of impairment of their cognitive functions. Such changes are not inevitable. To some extent, they can also be prevented.

Alzheimer's disease is widely recognised as the most common cause of dementia. Alzheimer's disease is not 'brain ageing'. It is an insidious disease which progresses slowly over 5 to 10 years. However, the degree of impairment in any one person with Alzheimer's may be quite variable in its severity and speed. Poor circulation to the brain makes it more likely that those with Alzheimer's will also develop dementia. This may be because the brain is very good at looking after itself, but it can only take so much.

The same process of progressive damage to blood vessels that leads to heart attacks and strokes in people with type 2 diabetes may also lead to a much more piecemeal loss of brain function. This is known as **vascular dementia** and is second only to Alzheimer's disease as a major cause of impaired cognitive function. As your brain uses over half of the body's glucose and at least 20 per cent of its oxygen, it is critically dependent on good blood flow. If blood supply is reduced to the brain, it turns down its activities, partly as a way of prolonging its survival. However, this may also be at the expense of its cognitive functions.

All the things that reduce your risk of stroke (detailed above) will also reduce your risk of dementia. Blood pressure lowering, sustained weight loss, improved glucose and lipid control, smoking cessation and regular physical activity can all help you retain your marbles.

There is also some evidence that the composition of your diet may also influence your risk of cognitive decline through its effects on your weight, blood pressure, glucose and lipid levels.

Diets high in trans fats and saturated (animal) fats are associated with faster rates of cognitive decline. By contrast, diets naturally high in fish and a Mediterranean diet high in monounsaturated fat (see Chapter 9) are associated with a lower risk of dementia. Maintaining a moderate level of regular physical activity is also associated with better preservation of the brain's functions.

Finally, it is also clear that regular mental activity is good for the brain. Any kind of social isolation can lead to mental stress, depression and mental decline. By contrast, remaining mentally challenged has a number of rewards, including keeping the brain sharp. There is no single answer for everyone. Some people will prefer solving crosswords to playing chess, bridge or Sudoku. Crafts, reading, learning new languages or skills can all be stimulating activities. It is possible to join a club or society and stay socially as well as mentally active. The trick is to find something challenging that you can enjoy every day to keep your brain active. This will also help to keep it healthy.

16.
Diabetes on my mood

UNDERSTAND

» It is perfectly normal to feel angry, guilty, overwhelmed, despondent, fearful or in denial about aspects of your diabetes.

» It is sometimes important to acknowledge and explore these feelings as a way to move forward.

» Stress is a killer and having diabetes is really stressful. This means that finding your own ways to deal with inevitable stresses is just as important as any other component of your diabetes care.

» Depression is a serious and common complication in people with type 2 diabetes.

» Depression is not a simple illness. It is sometimes difficult to see it for what it is against a background of other problems in people with type 2 diabetes.

MANAGE

» Cultivate your relationship with your diabetes care team. They will know what you are going through and have many resources available that can help.

» Don't shut off your emotions. They may be as much a determinant of your health as your diabetes is.

» Take the time to accent the positive and eliminate the negative in everything you do. Optimism is good for your health.
» Explore new ways to relax and unburden yourself.
» Recognise the symptoms of depression in yourself and ask for help in getting on top of them.

Effective management of diabetes is much more than biology and chemistry. It also means keeping your chin up and maintaining and optimising your mental wellbeing. This is not always easy.

Having diabetes is challenging. There are complex treatments, targets and goals, successes and failures. This often results in a range of emotional responses that are as different as the people who experience them. Broadly, these responses can be classified into eight different reactions:

1. **Anger and frustration**
   » 'Why me?'
   » 'It's not fair!'
   » 'How can this be happening to me?'
   » 'I hate my diabetes.'

2. **Denial/ridicule/rejection/disbelief**
   » 'I feel fine.'
   » 'This can't be happening to me.'
   » 'It's not that serious.'
   » 'It's only a touch of ...'

3. **Guilt/self-blame**
   » 'I caused this mess.'
   » 'It's all my fault.'
   » 'I deserved this.'

4. **Bargaining**
   » 'I have to do this now.'
   » 'If I do this, then ...'
   » 'I'll do anything for ...'
   » 'I don't care what it takes.'

5. **Withdrawal/nihilism/feeling overwhelmed/defeated/ fatigued/resigned/hopelessness**
   » 'It's all too hard.'
   » 'What's the point?'
   » 'Why should I bother to keep taking these/doing this?'
   » 'The harder I try the harder I fall.'
   » 'Stop the world I want to get off!'
   » 'I don't care any more.'

6. **Depression/negative thinking/low self-esteem**
   » 'I'm not worth the effort.'
   » 'They should just let me die.'
   » 'I'm stupid.'
   » 'I'm a bad person.'

7. **Stress/distress/anxiety/fear/dread**
   » 'What will happen now?'
   » 'What will I do if ...?'

8. **Acceptance**
   » 'I'm okay with my diabetes.'
   » 'I have a plan.'
   » 'It's just the way it is.'
   » 'I'll just have to get on with it.'

These different reactions are often called **defence** or **coping mechanisms**. They are perfectly normal. Part of coping with type 2 diabetes will inevitably involve experiencing some or all of these different emotional responses. They are not stages.

There is no particular order or requirement to experience any of these reactions. But at the same time, it is sometimes important to acknowledge and express these feelings as a way to move forward. You can also use these emotions as a trigger for change.

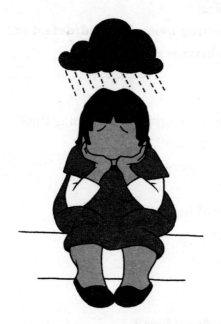

Having diabetes is challenging. This often results in a range of emotional responses that are as different as the people who experience them.

However, sometimes these emotions can get the better of you. This is often described as being 'stuck in a rut'. And this is when the stress of diabetes begins and when problems seem to magnify the longer you are stuck there. One of the most important differences between people who are able to survive their diabetes and those who succumb to its many challenges and complications lies in their ability to cope with illness and rebuild again and again.

Finding your way out is a personal journey, but one you shouldn't need to make alone. Your diabetes care team will know what you are going through and have many resources available that can help.

The best way to prevent stress from diabetes is to cultivate your relationship with your diabetes care team, and work with them to create and achieve common goals.

Some of the things they may get you to do include:

» *Disclosure.* Putting into words what you are feeling and letting others share your concerns can sometimes help you to know what you are really feeling. Talking to your diabetes management team, your family and friends will always make a difference. Even just communicating with yourself by keeping a personal diary can be a useful way to conceptualise your feelings.

» *Self-awareness.* Focus on the triggers that set you off. Find out what's making you angry or upset and when. Understand the things that make you feel good and find a way to go there when you're stuck.

» *Exploration.* Have a look at what other people with diabetes are experiencing. Read the blog or internet journal of someone else with type 2 diabetes. Attend group sessions where you hear about what other people are doing to keep control and how they are coping. Borrow new ideas or new recipes that might work for you.

» *Goal realignment.* Many of the challenges of diabetes come from unrealistic and unnecessary expectations. It is always important to realign your goals and aim to control what is in your control. This is where close contact with your diabetes management team will make a real difference and allow you to have a dynamic and evolving plan for coping with your diabetes.

» *Planning.* The best way to know where you should be going is to have a map. By establishing comprehensive plans and routines and following them closely, it is much easier to track your progress and never feel lost. Make your intensions clear to ensure you are in control of where your management is going. As you become more and more familiar with where you are, it also becomes easier to step off the map for brief periods and try new things, as you always know your way back.

» *Accenting the positive.* The impacts of any stress can be modified by changing the way it is perceived. If you think you are stressed, then you are. But when you think you have the resources to cope, then stress is no longer a threat. Some of this 'stress resilience' comes from confidence and coping skills. Some also comes from a positive outlook. All these can be cultivated and fostered. Stress-resilient people may have the same stressors (e.g. diabetes) but they expect everything will be okay, rather than a problem. They are better able to deal with stress because they know they can. A number of studies have shown that simply learning to 'accentuate the positive' in everything you do is associated with reduced stress and less heart disease. Optimism can be learned with practice and become part of your life.

Stress and its effect on diabetes

Every life is filled with many stresses. Your brain is the main driver of your response to stress, as well as its main target. It decides when there is a problem and acts automatically to gives the body the tools it needs to fight, survive or quickly run away (known as the 'fight or flight' response). The intensity of any stress response is determined not only by the perceived intensity of the threat, but also a host of other factors known cumulatively as your resilience (to stress). These include things like your genes, your gender, previous stressful experiences, coping skills and personality traits.

Having type 2 diabetes is a very stressful experience. Over and above your glucose control and any other aspect of your diabetes care, how you respond to this major stress in your life is also a major determinant of your subsequent health and wellbeing.

When stress gets the better of you it can cause many problems, including interfering with your ability to achieve and maintain control over them. In general, stressed people with type 2 diabetes have worse glucose control. This is not simply because they are too stressed to take their medication consistently or adhere to diet and lifestyle programs (although this doesn't help). The chemicals that are released in response to stress also serve to directly drive up glucose levels while at the same time limit the actions of insulin. At the same time, if you take people with type 2 diabetes and teach them yoga, meditation, tai chi or other relaxation techniques, on average you will achieve improvements in their glucose control roughly equivalent to adding in an additional glucose-lowering medication.

Over and above its effect on your glucose control, chronic activation of the stress response can also increase your risk of complications from your diabetes, including:

» *Heart attacks and strokes.* Up to one-third of all heart attacks may be attributable to chronic stress. For example, people reporting stress at work or marital stress have twice the risk of having a heart attack or stroke. This increase in risk due to stress is about the same as having a high cholesterol level or being a smoker.

» *High blood pressure.* In susceptible people (especially those with diabetes), stress can drive the blood pressure higher. By contrast, effective stress management invariably lowers blood pressure and improves the function of blood vessels.

» *Infections.* When you are stressed you seem to pick up every bug that is going around. Stress also reduces the effectiveness of vaccination to diseases like the flu. These are just some examples of the effects that stress can have on your ability to fight off infections. Of course in diabetes, when your immunity is low anyway, stress is the last thing you need.

» *Brain function.* Any stress can make it difficult to concentrate, learn and focus. But prolonged stress will actually cause some areas of the brain to shrink.

» *Depression and mental illness.* In certain susceptible individuals, chronic stress can trigger depression (see below) and other mental illnesses.

» *Sleep.* Stress can interfere with you getting the sleep you need each night. This can lead to even more stress (see Chapter 17).

» *Sexual function.* Stress can also interfere with your sex life (see Chapter 18).

One important way to cope with having diabetes is to manage your (inevitable) stress better. Some people will need more help than others, based on their resilience and the size of their burden. But everyone will need some help sooner or later.

There are many different ways you can handle stress: some you can do yourself (also known as self-help programs) and others you perform with the help of different health practitioners. Some of the most well-known and effective stress management techniques include relaxation, mind–body techniques, mindful breathing, biofeedback, hypnosis, yoga, tai chi, exercise, mindfulness meditation, guided imagery, conditioning, and time out. Gardening or listening to music can be equally effective. When used routinely, each serves to build resilience to stress in some people. But it's not the same for everyone. Not everyone can do yoga. Not everyone likes gardening. The most effective strategies are the ones you enjoy, the ones that put your mind at ease and the ones you want to do again and again.

There are many drugs that can also be useful in some people suffering from severe and chronic stress. Each one has its side effects and limitations. In addition, most lose their effectiveness in the long term, especially on their own. The combination with other stress management techniques better allows these chemicals to be used for only short periods, when the stress is most acute, with other techniques coming into their own once control is achieved.

Depression and diabetes

Depression is a serious and common problem for people with type 2 diabetes. It is common for everyone to feel low at times during their life. But depression is a disproportionate and pervasive mood that interferes with your ability to function. It can affect your relationships, your work, your sleep and many other aspects of your health and wellbeing. Depression can also affect your diabetes control, the likelihood of complications and their impact.

Not everyone with diabetes will become depressed, no matter how bad their illness gets. Certainly, women are twice as likely to become depressed as men. Single people are more at risk than married ones. At the same time those people who stay socially connected with their family and friends have a lower risk of depression.

Depression is not a simple illness. It is sometimes difficult to see it for what it is against a background of other problems in people with type 2 diabetes. However, identifying and managing depression is an important and under-recognised part of diabetes care.

One way to identify those people who could be depressed is the Patient Health Questionnaire-2. It asks only two simple questions:

1. Have you often had little interest or pleasure in doing things over the past month?
2. Have you often been bothered by feeling down, depressed or hopeless over the past month?

Most people suffering from depression will answer yes to one or both of these questions. If this is you, then it is worth talking to your doctor or other members of your diabetes care team about the need for further evaluation. About half of those with positive responses will turn out not to be depressed, but it is still important to ask your doctor or specialist for their formal assessment.

Treating depression

Depression is not something you have to put up with. Like any other illness, depression can be treated. Not only will this make you feel and function better, the effective treatment of depression will also mean better diabetes control.

A number of different treatment options are available that will be suited to different people and different clinical situations. Most doctors will often first try to use treatments that don't involve taking pills. The most widely used of these is **psychotherapy** (also known as counselling). This can be very effective in many people with depression. The response rate is roughly similar to that of taking antidepressant pills, although when combined they may be even more effective than either alone.

There are many different forms of psychotherapy, but most involve structured weekly sessions delivered by trained therapists to retrain thinking and behaviour or develop new coping skills. Relaxation and stress management are also key components. These sessions can be delivered to you alone or as part of a group.

Participation in **physical exercise programs**, or increasing your physical activity in a social setting (such as walking the dog, golf, walking groups, tennis, etc.), can also significantly improve symptoms of depression in some people and have a range of other benefits for your overall health (see Chapter 5).

Many people with depression also need **antidepressant** pills to help them out. Each of these medications acts in a different way to balance disturbed chemistry in the depressed brain. Medications include:

» Selective serotonin-reuptake inhibitors (SSRIs). These are often used as the first-line drug treatment for depression, especially in those over 60.

» Serotonin–norepinephrine reuptake inhibitors (SNRIs). These may be particularly useful for patients with chronic pain due to nerve damage associated with diabetes.

» Tricyclic antidepressants (TCAs). These agents are effective but may have significant side effects, especially in those with heart problems.

» Monoamine oxidase inhibitors (MAOIs). These older agents also work in some patients, but require close monitoring and a special diet to prevent side effects, so may be less suitable for those with type 2 diabetes.

Antidepressants do not blunt normal emotional reactions or turn you into a zombie. Antidepressants also do not lead to dependence or addiction. However, many of these medications do have significant side effects, so are used only where having depression is a worse alternative.

About half of those treated with any given antidepressant show a positive response, often within as little as a month of treatment, although it may take a few more months for a full response to occur. Once a remission is achieved, antidepressants are usually continued for a further 6 to 12 months, as stopping too soon can increase the risk of recurrence. In those who do not respond initially, a trial of an alternative antidepressant or combination of medicines, with or without psychotherapy, is often undertaken. Where needed, the actions of antidepressants can sometimes be augmented by other medications, such as lithium or anticonvulsants.

There are a number of different supplements and over-the-counter herbal remedies that are advertised to help treat the symptoms of depression in some people. However, their effectiveness is variable, and most people experience little or no benefit from them.

17

Diabetes in my sleep

UNDERSTAND

- » Good quality sleep in good quantities is important for daytime health and wellbeing.
- » Sleep problems are a common complication of type 2 diabetes, yet often go unrecognised against a background of other issues.
- » Cramps and restless legs are not something you simply have to put up with because you have type 2 diabetes.
- » Obstructive sleep apnoea affects at least one-quarter of people with type 2 diabetes, especially men and those who are overweight.

MANAGE

- » Ask your partner about how you are sleeping, whether you are snoring or waking often with a start.
- » Make changes to your bedroom and night routines that will help you get the sleep you need.
- » Aim to control your glucose levels during the night as well as the day.
- » Don't let your bladder get in the way of a good night's sleep. There are a number of simple ways to retrain your bladder and make it less irritable.

A good night's sleep is an important part of a healthy life. The third of your life you spend asleep can significantly affect the two-thirds you spend awake. Everyone needs a good quantity of sleep and good quality sleep to keep their brain and body working in peak condition. This is especially the case in those with type 2 diabetes.

Sleep serves a number of essential functions you simply can't do without. It does far more than just passively conserve your energy for daytime activities.

Without sleep you not only feel tired, but many other things don't work, including your attempts to successfully manage your diabetes.

There is good evidence to show that too little sleep, and in particular too little quality sleep, can contribute to a range of problems:

» Excessive weight gain. Those with habitually poor sleep tend to gain weight more easily and struggle to take it off. This is partly explained by the fact that tired bodies think they have too little energy and try to compensate by making you feel hungry, encouraging you to eat more. This is the last thing someone with type 2 diabetes really needs.

» Poor glucose control. Those with habitually poor sleep often have difficulty achieving and maintaining control of blood glucose levels. In fact, poor sleep is actually associated with an increased risk for developing type 2 diabetes.

» Higher blood pressure and cholesterol levels.

» Irregular heart rhythms, including atrial fibrillation, a risk factor for strokes (see Chapter 15).

» Increased risk of errors in judgement, loss of performance and accidents, especially from falling asleep while driving.

» Low mood, motivation and energy.

» Increased sensitivity to pain.

» Reduced resistance to infection.

Sleep also significantly affects the building of your memories. Your body may be resting when you're asleep, but this allows your brain to get on with the important task of processing your day. During deep sleep the brain rewires its circuits to make lasting connections between events, sensations and other information. This is called **consolidation**. It ensures that all newly gained knowledge is organised and stored for future use. Getting more quality sleep really does help you remember, process and understand things better. This is partly why the ability to think and process in the daytime declines the less sleep you get (not just because you feel tired). This is also why an active brain demands more sleep, like those of children and adolescents.

However, the most important consequence of too little night-time sleep is daytime sleepiness! Everyone has been through those exhausted days where you have difficulty concentrating, remembering and feel generally moody and irritable. It's easy to know what the answer is. You can't wait to just go home and go to bed! However, small amounts of sleep debt can creep up on you. And after a period of missing too much sleep, stress takes over the show, increasing blood pressure and producing stress hormones, which also make it even harder for you to sleep.

What is sleep?

Most people think of sleep as a continuous loss of consciousness that lasts for 7 to 9 hours every night. In fact, the normal sleep pattern is more like a roller-coaster ride. After going to bed, you usually fall asleep within about 15 to 30 minutes. You spend a few minutes in very light sleep then slowly descend into deeper and deeper sleep. This deep sleep is the most important for rejuvenating you for the next day, and brain activity during this deep sleep is characterised by delta waves. This is the same activity induced by meditation.

After about an hour, you ascend into lighter sleep and about 10 minutes later enter the phase known as rapid eye movement (REM) sleep during which your brain is very active. This is when you have most of your dreams, and your eyes are darting around as if watching an action movie. After about 20 minutes, your brain falls asleep and the roller-coaster ride of sleep starts all over again.

The whole sleep cycle takes about an hour and a half. REM sleep accounts for about 20 to 25 per cent of the time you are asleep, and deep (non-REM) sleep accounts for the other 75 to 80 per cent. The proportion of each sleep cycle spent in deep sleep tends to be greater in the first cycles of the night, while REM sleep tends to be longer in the later cycles, so that by the final sleep cycle of the night you spend approximately half your sleep cycle (dreaming) in REM sleep.

If one cycle is cut short in any component of your sleep (such as when you drink alcohol, which suppresses REM sleep), you tend to catch up in others (so that when the booze wears off the morning dreams are longer and more vivid on the rebound).

Most people fit in about five cycles a night. It is quite normal to wake out of your light sleep in between your sleep cycles. In fact this becomes quite common as sleep becomes lighter as people get older. Being awake at some time during the night is not a sign of problems with your sleep and is not something to stay awake worrying about. Historical records suggest that our ancestors probably used to sleep in two parts: an initial sleep of around 4 to 5 hours (three sleep cycles) followed by 1 to 2 hours of being awake and then a second sleep period of another 3 hours (another two sleep cycles).

How do you know you are getting enough?

The amount of quality sleep you need for good health is hard to define. There is no magic number of hours that suits everyone. Some people need 9 hours yet others function very well on 6 hours' sleep.

The amount of sleep needed varies from person to person as well as varying for the same person at different stages of their life.

The amount of sleep you need also varies through the seasons and even over the course of the working week. One simple way to tell if you're getting sufficient sleep is that you should feel refreshed and able to function throughout the day.

If you are waking up still tired and lethargic or if you habitually doze off or fall asleep through the day, it may be that you are not getting the sleep you need. Of course, there may be other reasons apart from poor sleep for not feeling your best through the day, so talk to your doctor about what the next step should be (and certainly before starting to treat yourself). To see if poor sleep is really your problem, your doctor will also often ask you to keep a sleep diary, to find out just how much sleep you are really getting and how it affects your life during the day.

Most people suffer from trouble sleeping at some time during their lives. But this is usually short-lived and settles on its own with no lasting effects. However, it is clear that people who are habitually sleeping less than 6 hours night after night have an increased risk of problems with their health, including diabetes. Similarly, those who report habitually broken sleep or difficulty staying asleep for long periods through the night appear to have more problems with their health.

Interestingly, those people who usually sleep more than 10 hours a night also have more health problems. This may reflect their broken sleep pattern, lack of quality sleep and desperate need to catch up.

How might diabetes affect your sleep?

Having diabetes can impact on your nights as much as your days. It can stop you getting the sleep you need in a number of different ways.

Diabetes can indirectly affect your sleep pattern by causing you to need to get up and go to the toilet, often many times during the night. This is known as **nocturia**. Healthy kidneys are able to make more concentrated urine overnight. This means that most adults do not need to get up more than once, if at all. However, getting up more frequently at night is a common symptom of diabetes and a common cause of disrupted sleep.

Nocturia can sometimes be a sign of poor glucose control during the night. When glucose levels get too high, glucose spills over into your urine, which increases the amount of urine you will make (see Chapter 14). This is most noticeable at night, when you should normally be making less. Most people don't test their glucose levels at night (as they are asleep) so it can be hard to detect. But when glucose control is improved, this symptom can quickly go away. So it is always worthwhile pointing it out to your diabetes care team and asking their advice.

Damage to the kidneys or the bladder associated with diabetes may also cause you to get up frequently in the night. Many people with type 2 diabetes benefit from bladder retraining and/or taking medications in the evening to reduce the irritability of their bladder. These are discussed in detail in Chapter 14.

Passing more urine at night can also be a sign of problems

with your heart. Again, instead of making less urine during the night, some people with impaired heart function (known as heart failure) make more. This is to enable them to clear the extra fluid from their body that has accumulated in their legs during the day, but comes back into their system when they lie down. This is treated by diuretics — medication to increase the amount of fluid lost into the urine through the day, making less of a burden at night.

Sometimes, low glucose levels (hypoglycaemia) at night can also cause you to wake up. To protect against hypoglycaemia, the body has a number of defence mechanisms that trigger warning symptoms to alert you that things are awry. One of them is to wake you up and make it hard to go back to sleep until you have eaten. Again, hypos can't occur in the majority of people with type 2 diabetes because their body is able to make enough glucose in the event that levels fall. However, in some people with type 2 diabetes who take medications that increase their insulin levels (sulphonylureas and meglitinides) or are injecting insulin itself, hypos can occur at night. Techniques for avoiding and treating hypos are discussed in detail in Chapter 7.

Type 2 diabetes is also associated with increased levels of stress and mental illness, including depression and anxiety disorders. These can significantly affect the quantity and quality of your sleep. Their assessment and management are discussed in the previous chapter.

The health of your feet also affects how well you sleep. It is not unusual for people with type 2 diabetes to experience pain in their feet (due to ulcers, infection, nerve damage and/or vascular disease). Pain from these foot problems is often worse at night (or even limited to night-time) as the feet are elevated, warm and partly compressed by the bedclothes. These conditions are discussed in detail in Chapter 12. Each has a specific treatment that includes medication and/or surgery; in addition, simple things such as using a bed cradle can keep sheets and blankets from touching your sensitive feet and legs.

Some people with type 2 diabetes experience an unpleasant 'crawling' feeling in their legs at night, accompanied by a tremendous urge to move. This is known as **restless legs syndrome**. It is often dismissed as something due to your diabetes, back problems or 'just nerves'. However, a number of different medications are now available to tackle this real problem, once it is recognised for what it is.

Another problem that can keep you up at night is **leg cramps**, usually affecting the calves but also sometimes the thighs or the feet. These cramps can be intensely painful and last up to several minutes before subsiding. This is followed by a deep muscle ache that can last up to a few hours. Leg cramps are more common in people with type 2 diabetes, especially older people, those with kidney problems or poor circulation. Again, this is not a problem that should be simply put up with. In those with troubling or frequent cramping, symptoms can be reduced by using verapamil or diltaizem (commonly prescribed as blood pressure-lowering medications). Vitamin B complex may also be helpful in some people. Quinine, the active ingredient in tonic water, may also be useful in some people although its effects are quite variable.

Snoring and obstructive sleep apnoea

Some people with type 2 diabetes experience sudden episodes of shortness of breath and/or coughing at night (known as **paroxysms**) which wake them from their sleep. These episodes

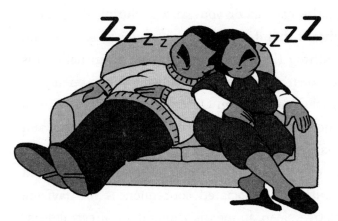

Everyone snores at some time in their life. However, those with type 2 diabetes snore much more frequently and loudly.

can have a number of different causes, including heart and kidney problems (see chapters 10 and 13). However, one of the most common and important causes is a condition called **obstructive sleep apnoea**, in which the flow of air becomes temporarily blocked while you are deeply asleep, causing you to choke for a brief moment before the act of waking up opens your airway and allows the air to flow freely again.

When you fall deeply asleep, your body goes into a floppy state of relaxation. This also happens in your airway. Like sucking through a straw, the 'suck' of air associated with breathing causes your (now floppy) airway to cave in a little bit when you are asleep. This happens in everyone when they sleep. But if your airway is already narrowed or is excessively floppy, it can get very tight. Often this makes the normally smooth flow of air into the lungs become turbulent. Like sucking air through a narrow straw, this is noisy and is heard by others as **snoring**.

Everyone snores at some time in their life, such as when you have a cold, when your throat is swollen, or when you (and your airways) are excessively relaxed when drunk or using sleeping pills. However, those with type 2 diabetes, especially those who are very overweight, snore much more frequently and loudly.

Sometimes, the cave-in of your airway during deep sleep can be so significant that it completely obstructs all air flow and stops your breathing (known as an **apnoea**). Eventually, this wakes you up (known as an **arousal**), allowing you to open your airway and breathe freely again. Obstructive sleep apnoea is a condition that occurs when this cycle of obstruction, apnoea and arousal happens over and over again during every sleep (more than five times every hour). This results in a very fragmented sleep pattern with the associated consequences on daytime health. Obstructive sleep apnoea is thought to affect at least one-quarter of people with type 2 diabetes.

These sudden dramatic arousals through the night don't just break up your sleep. The release of stress hormones with each episode can also drive up glucose, blood pressure and lipid levels. This may contribute to an increased risk of heart disease and strokes in snorers.

It is hard to know you have obstructive sleep apnoea. Luckily, partners or family members will often complain about your loud snoring with periods of silence followed by gasps, choking episodes or sudden arousals. Without the help of these observations you may just be feeling excessively tired or inattentive during the daytime. This could have many causes and your sleep pattern gets overlooked as a cause of daytime issues. Once it is suspected, it is very easy to find out whether obstructive sleep apnoea is present by using a **sleep test**. During this simple test your breathing pattern is observed while you are sleeping.

There are now a number of treatments for obstructive sleep apnoea that differ depending on the severity of the problem and the presence of other medical problems. For people with type 2 diabetes, the most important treatment is losing weight through diet, exercise and, if necessary, bariatric surgery (see Chapter 4).

Simple manoeuvres such as avoiding alcohol and sleeping pills (which relax an already narrow airway), quitting smoking or sleeping on your side can also reduce snoring and apnoeas. Sleeping at a 30-degree angle, in a recliner chair or adjustable bed, can also be effective, especially in very overweight people. Special exercises to strengthen the muscles of the airways can also help. One of these useful exercises includes getting men to learn to play the didgeridoo (for cultural reasons it should not be played by women). Special dental splints can also be used to hold open the airway. These look similar to mouthguards used in sport to protect the teeth. When properly fitted, a dental splint will reduce snoring and help in mild to moderate cases of obstructive sleep apnoea.

For severe cases, the most effective way to reduce sleepiness and other daytime impacts is **continuous positive airway pressure (CPAP)**. This means sleeping with a facemask that blows pressurised air into your airways to hold them open, just as the pressure of air in a balloon keeps it expanded. Not everyone can tolerate CPAP because of discomfort, noise, congestion or claustrophobia. But for those who can, it can lead to weight loss, improved mood and overall health.

Getting a good night's sleep

Problems with your sleep are typically chronic and do not go away by themselves. Each of the ways in which diabetes disrupts your sleep can be effectively managed in conjunction with your diabetes care team. Treating the underlying condition may resolve some or many of your symptoms. However, it may not necessarily improve your sleep. While fixing these other problems increases the chances that your sleep will improve, treating both your sleep and other conditions that influence it can simultaneously improve the outcomes for each.

Just because sleep is an unconscious activity doesn't mean you have no control over it.

The things you do while you're awake can greatly influence the quality and quantity of your sleep.

There are a number of simple things you can do to make it easier to get the sleep you need. These are known collectively as **sleep hygiene**. In essence, these activities accent the positive triggers that help you to go to sleep while eliminating many of the negative barriers that serve to keep you awake.

» *Darkness.* Keep your bedroom dark. Block out the light from the street or the next room.

» *Coolness.* Falling body temperature is an important cue for bedtime and sleep. This can be enhanced by keeping your bedroom cooler than the rest of the house, or by having a bath or shower in the evening, allowing natural cooling to enhance your sleep.

» *Quiet.* Noise and stimulation are supposed to keep us awake. The bedroom should therefore be a quiet place.

» *Routine.* Most people establish a routine for their night-time activities. When this is disrupted, so is their sleep. For those with trouble sleeping it is sometimes useful to establish a pattern of going to bed and waking at the same time every day, even on weekends. Go to bed when your body tells you you're sleepy and get up when you wake. Bright sunlight in the morning also helps to regulate your body clock.

» *Comfort.* Your bed should be a comfortable place. You spend more of your lifetime there than any other single place. But beds seldom receive as much attention as the car or the television. Simple things can help, such as replacing your worn out, uneven or uncomfortable mattress and pillows with those that allow you to maintain an anatomically neutral position. Keeping the pressure off your feet with a cradle or a short quilt can also be helpful for sleep.

» *No stimulation.* The brain is supposed to be winding down for sleep. Taking caffeine (in tea or coffee) any time after 2 p.m. can see the buzz staying around until bedtime. Similarly, late meals can keep the brain going; late-night snacks are not a long-term solution for hypoglycaemia (see Chapter 7). Also, keep the television and the computer out of the bedroom, as both of these keep the eyes and the mind active when you should be sleeping.

There are a number of short-term interventions for insomnia, including the use of **sleeping pills** (also known as **sedatives**). These can help reestablish a pattern and restore confidence that a good night's sleep is achievable. However, using sleeping pills may be associated with side effects, including residual daytime sleepiness and dependence if used chronically. A number of psychological (training) techniques can also help sleep in the short term, with far fewer side effects.

18.
Diabetes in my bed

UNDERSTAND

» While diabetes does not prevent sex, it can sometimes reduce the ability to achieve satisfying and enjoyable sex.

» For women with type 2 diabetes the most common sexual problem is a low libido.

» Women with diabetes may also find it difficult to attain adequate vaginal lubrication, making intercourse uncomfortable and climax more difficult to reach.

» For men with type 2 diabetes, the most common problem is an inability to get or maintain an erection. This may affect up to three-quarters of all men with type 2 diabetes.

MANAGE

» Be honest with yourself and your partner. Pretending that there is no problem is not a solution.

» Ask for help. There are many safe and effective medical treatments now available which, alongside psychological support, can help you to rediscover your sex life.

» Change the way you approach sex to be more in keeping with what your body can do. More foreplay, more stimulation and more lubrication are all practical and enjoyable additions that will help make sex work better for you.

The bed is not just for sleep. For many people, sex is a major part of their health, wellbeing, self-esteem and quality of life. It is often said that sex keeps you alive. This is more than just having the kind of relationship or youthful vigour that makes frequent sex possible. Satisfying sex seems to be associated with better health. It also serves to enhance intimacy and reinforce relationships. By contrast, when sex becomes a let-down it can not only be frustrating but it can also be harmful for your health.

While diabetes does not prevent sex, it can sometimes reduce the ability to achieve satisfying and enjoyable sex. This is known as sexual dysfunction.

Dealing with a low libido

Desire for or interest in sex is known as **libido**. Having a low libido is a common sexual issue for many people with type 2 diabetes. A number of different factors may be involved. A low libido can be the result of complex changes in brain and body chemistry due to diabetes. Equally, psychological factors such as physical fatigue, body image, pain, poor sleep, low self-esteem and stress can make sex the last thing on your mind.

There is good evidence that keeping good control of your glucose levels will also help you keep your sex life going. But for those who are experiencing problems in bed, better glucose control is not enough. Helping you find your libido again usually involves working with your mind as well as your body. It cannot be fixed by taking medications such as Viagra, which only work on the penis.

There are many valuable practitioners who can discreetly assist couples and help to put them back on the right track. Some of the most successful treatments are delivered by sex therapists, who work on improving a couple's closeness and communication both in and out of the bedroom through guided discussion, getting rid of negative thoughts and unrealistic performance goals.

In some people, type 2 diabetes may be the cause of reduced levels of sex hormones such as **testosterone**. This can contribute to a reduced desire for sex both in men and women. Low testosterone levels can also cause you to feel tired, reduce your capacity to concentrate and disturb your sleep. Note that not everyone with low testosterone levels will have problems with their health or need to be treated. But in those people with low levels who are also experiencing troublesome symptoms, taking hormone supplements can improve how they feel both in the bedroom and out of it.

For men, there are a range of different testosterone supplements that can be prescribed, including injections, patches and gels. The best one for you will be determined by specific blood tests, which will confirm that your levels are low and allow your doctor to develop an individualised treatment plan. In post-menopausal women with low testosterone levels, only small doses may be required to restore normal levels and improve energy and libido. This can often be simply achieved by taking chemicals such as DHEA, which are partly metabolised into testosterone.

In each case, these supplements work best for restoring a flagging libido when combined with psychological support and good diabetes management. Taking testosterone or DHEA is seldom enough on its own to bring sex back into your life.

A number of over-the-counter medications advertise their ability to increase sexual desire. This is largely because people think they do. But because sexual desire is mostly in the mind it probably doesn't matter. However, their safety and the consistency of their effects may be quite variable.

Diabetes and the vagina

Some women with type 2 diabetes may also find it difficult to attain adequate **vaginal lubrication**, making intercourse uncomfortable and climax more difficult to reach. Vaginal dryness is a common problem in women with type 2 diabetes due to fluid losses that also cause the eyes and the mouth to feel dry. But even in those with good glucose control, dryness may be a symptom of hormonal changes associated with diabetes or damage to the blood vessels and nerves of the pelvis. Some medications used to treat diabetes can also reduce vaginal lubrication. It is also a frequent complaint of ageing.

Although common, this need not be a barrier to sexual enjoyment. It just needs to be recognised and so incorporated into how you have sex. For example, all women with diabetes will benefit from sufficient stimulation/foreplay to ensure that lubrication is naturally enhanced before sex. The use of lubricants can also help and form a new fun part of sex. Oestrogen-containing creams can improve the health of the vagina and its ability to make lubricating fluids during sex. However, hormone replacement therapy is not appropriate for post-menopausal women with type 2 diabetes because of the increased risk of heart disease and clotting.

Women with type 2 diabetes are also prone to genital infections, especially thrush. This can be quite uncomfortable and distressing. Although thrush is easily treated, it is common for it to come back repeatedly and further courses of treatment are often needed. Achieving and maintaining good glucose control will reduce your chances of getting thrush and assist in its eradication. Other tricks to prevent thrush include oestrogen creams which help to build your resistance to infection. Probiotic bacteria, such as lactobacilli in yoghurt and some supplements, may also help to prevent infection in some cases.

Not getting an erection

It's perfectly normal for men to have an occasional problem keeping an erection. But for some men, these difficulties are frequent and severe, making sex all but impossible.

A consistent inability to get or maintain an erection for sex is the most common sexual problem affecting men with type 2 diabetes.

This is known as **erectile dysfunction** and may affect at least three-quarters of men with type 2 diabetes. An inability to maintain an erection can be the result of many factors. Coordinated function among nerves and blood vessels and the right mindset are all required for the penis to become and stay erect. If any of these necessary components isn't functioning optimally, an erection will fail. Unfortunately, type 2 diabetes can affect all these different components, which is why erectile dysfunction is so common.

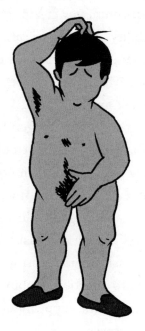

The consistent inability to get or maintain an erection may affect over three-quarters of men with type 2 diabetes. But this can be fixed!

The good news is that there are a number of very effective treatments now available. The most widely used treatments are the type 5 phosphodiesterase inhibitors, the first and most well known of which is **Viagra**. There are also now many others available that vary in how long they work for. This influences when they need to be taken before sex and how long they last. Viagra is usually taken about an hour before sex and lasts for around 8 hours. Some other medications can be taken many hours before and still work a day later.

These pills work by increasing blood flow to the penis when it is stimulated, enhancing the chances of an erection. These medications have no direct effect on the penis in the absence of sexual stimulation, so won't cause an erection unless you want one. However, they work in only about 60 per cent of men with type 2 diabetes.

Viagra has no direct effect on your mind so it won't make you suddenly sex crazed. However, it does have a profound psychological effect that comes from the anticipation of sex. Viagra and other medications of the same class are generally safe. Some men experience headaches, flushing or nasal stuffiness. They shouldn't be used in people with heart problems requiring nitroglycerine as part of their treatment.

An alternative to pills are penis injections or tiny suppositories placed inside the penis. These act to trigger an erection within 10 to 15 minutes whenever they are used. Unlike Viagra, they produce erections without any stimulation so are helpful in people with diabetes who have nerve damage. Because they only act in your groin they have few side effects elsewhere. The erection usually subsides within an hour. Other options include vacuum erection devices and penile prostheses. When used in the right setting, each can improve sex and your quality of life.

Always ask for help

While dissatisfaction with sex is common in both men and women with type 2 diabetes, it is not the first thing you hear people complain about when they see their diabetes care team. Just focusing on glucose control sometimes means that you are not focusing on your total health and wellbeing. Ignoring the problem does not make it go away and can sometimes make it worse.

The biggest barrier is usually a reluctance to share your feelings, and reticence in asking for help from your partner or your health specialist. Sex and sexuality are often kept too private. It is not that you don't know there is a problem. Rather, most people are understandably uncomfortable disclosing or discussing sexual matters. Yet there are many effective resources now available to prevent diabetes coming in the way of a healthy and fulfilling sex life. This always means first asking for help.

Acknowledgements

Baker IDI would like to thank Professor Don Chisholm AO, Garvan Institute of Medical Research; Dr Pat Phillips, Endocrinologist, The QE Specialist Centre, Woodville, South Australia; and Professor Trisha Dunning AM, Chair in Nursing and Director Centre for Nursing and Allied Health Research Deakin University and Barwon Health, who provided insightful and independent reviews of the early draft text.

We would also like to acknowledge the following Baker IDI staff: Professor Mark Cooper, Associate Professor Jonathan Shaw, Ms Michele Mack and Ms Rebecca Stiegler, who provided their time and expertise in reviewing the book.

The generosity of these reviewers has helped to create a text that is accurate, useful and understandable to readers.

Resources

There are many pages on the internet to help you learn more about type 2 diabetes. Here are some good sites to get you started. There are many more you'll be able to discover as you continue to explore your diabetes and its treatment. Just be careful, as some make claims that cannot be supported. Always discuss possible changes in your management with your diabetes care team before embarking on them and never use them to the exclusion of your recommended treatment.

The Baker IDI Heart and Diabetes Institute

http://www.bakeridi.edu.au/Diabetes_Resources_Fact_Sheets/

By the author

http://www.bakeridi.edu.au/research/biochemistry_of_diabetic_complications/

http://www.slowageingbook.com

http://www.penguin.com.au/products/9780143202264/csiro-and-baker-idi-diabetes-diet-and-lifestyle-plan

Diabetes organisations

http://www.cdc.gov/diabetes/consumer/index.htm

http://www.diabetesaustralia.com.au

http://www.diabetes.ca/

http://www.diabeteschannel.com.au

http://www.diabetes.co.uk/

http://www.diabetes.org

http://www.diabetes.org.nz/resources/pamphlets

http://www.iddt.org/

http://www.idf.org/
http://ndep.nih.gov/i-have-diabetes/index.aspx

Diet

http://www.diabetes-book.com/index.shtml
http://www.diabetes-diet.org.uk/
http://diabeticmediterraneandiet.com/
http://www.dsolve.com/
http://www.glycemicindex.com
http://www.gofor2and5.com.au
http://lowcarbdiabetic.co.uk/
http://myphotodiet.com/
http://www.nhs.uk/Change4Life

Exercise

http://www.10000steps.org.au
http://www.diabeticlifestyle.com/exercise/diabetes-beginning-exercise-plan
http://www.getwalking.org/
http://www.liftforlife.com.au
http://www.runsweet.com/

Complications

http://www.beyondblue.org.au
http://diabetespeptalk.ca/en/
http://www.hearthub.org/
http://www.heartfoundation.org.au
http://www.kidney.org
http://www.kidney.org.au
http://www.limbs4life.com/
http://www.nei.nih.gov/health/diabetic/retinopathy.asp

OTHER USEFUL DIABETES RESOURCES AND BLOGS

http://www.battlediabetes.com/

http://www.bbc.co.uk/health/physical_health/conditions/in_
depth/diabetes/index.shtml

http://www.diabetesandrelatedhealthissues.com/

http://diabetes.boomja.com/

http://www.diabetescare.net/

http://www.diabetesdigest.com/

http://DiabetesEveryDay.com

http://www.diabetesforum.com/

http://www.diabeteshealth.com/

http://www.diabeteslocal.org/

http://www.diabetesmine.com/

http://www.diabetesmonitor.com/

http://www.diabeteswellbeing.com/

http://www.irunoninsulin.com/

http://www.mydiabetesmyway.scot.nhs.uk/default.asp

http://www.patient.co.uk/education/diabetes

http://www.thediabetesresource.com/

Index

EXISLE
PUBLISHING

e-newsletter

If you value books like we do why not subscribe to our e-newsletter? As a subscriber you'll receive special offers and discounts, be the first to hear of our exciting upcoming titles & be kept up to date with book tours and author events. You'll also receive unique opportunities exclusive to subscribers — and much more.

To subscribe in Australia or from all other countries except New Zealand visit:
www.exislepublishing.com.au/newsletter-sign-up
For New Zealand visit:
www.exislepublishing.co.nz/newsletter-subscribe